※ the hugely better calorie counter

essentials

✳ the hugely better calorie counter

essentials

carolyn humphries

foulsham

LONDON • NEW YORK • TORONTO • SYDNEY

foulsham

The Publishing House, Bennetts Close, Cippenham, Slough, Berkshire, SL1 5AP, England

ISBN 0-572-02754-0

Neither the editors of W. Foulsham & Co. Ltd nor the author nor the publisher take responsibility for any possible consequences from any procedure, test, exercise or action by any person reading or following the information in this book. The publication of this book does not constitute the practice of medicine, and this book does not attempt to replace any diet or instructions from your doctor. The author and publisher advise the reader to check with a doctor before starting a diet, administering any medication or undertaking any course of treatment or exercise.

Printed in Great Britain by Cox & Wyman, Reading, Berkshire

Contents

Introduction

There are lots of calorie counters in the bookshops, but this one is, I think, genuinely different – and hugely better. Before starting to write it, I thought very carefully about how you want to *use* a calorie counter. Having looked at those already on offer, I asked myself some questions.

- Is it useful to have to search for things under obscure brand names where you can't find them and can't compare them easily with similar products? No!

- Do you want to work out what category a food belongs to before you even try to find it? Hardly likely.

- Do you really have time to worry that one Rich Tea biscuit has four more calories than another? I don't think so.

- Is it helpful to tell you the calories per 100 g, leaving you to work out how much you are eating and how many calories it contains? Do you really want to carry a kitchen scales and a calculator when you're going to meet your friends in that hot new café? Life's too short!

With this handy little book you can forget all of those problems, because it gives you the real essentials, uniquely organised and calculated to make everything easy. It tells you how many calories you are consuming in everything you eat, from breakfast through to dinner – every snack and every drink, at home or eating out.

Most people who use this book will be doing so because they want to lose weight, but you can also use it if you want to gain weight. It may be small, but this at-a-glance calorie and nutrient ready-reckoner has all the information you need to achieve and maintain a healthy lifestyle, including great tips that really will make dieting easy.

A Healthy Lifestyle

Dieting of any kind, whether to lose or gain weight, should be part of a healthy lifestyle. Crank dieting is stupid and it doesn't work. If you try to lose weight by cutting out a particular food group, you may succeed, but you'll also become unfit and possibly even ill. In the same way, if you are trying to gain weight, eating mountains of sugary and fatty foods is not the answer.

Your body needs nutrients containing vitamins and minerals as well as the proper balance of protein, carbohydrate, fat and fibre to keep you fit and healthy. So as well as the calories, this book gives you the amounts of each of these food groups per portion of each food. With this information you can see which foods are good sources of which nutrient, and so ensure that you have the correct proportions each day.

Proteins

Your body needs protein to maintain good health and to repair itself when necessary. The best sources of proteins are fish, lean meat, poultry, dairy products, eggs and vegetable proteins such as pulses (dried peas, beans and lentils), tofu and Quorn. Eat two to three small portions a day.

Carbohydrates

It may surprise you to know that carbohydrates, or starchy foods, should make up 50 per cent of each of your meals. This is because complex carbohydrates provide us with energy and are vital to our well-being. However, the sugar (simple carbohydrates) and fat you mix with them will pile on the unwanted calories that can harm your health. The best sources are bread (all types), pasta, rice, cereals (this includes breakfast cereals but you should choose wholegrain varieties not sugar-coated ones) and potatoes. Eat plenty of all of these.

Vitamins and minerals

These are also essential for general good health. The best sources are fruit and vegetables. They should, preferably, be fresh, but frozen or canned in water or natural juice with no added sugar (and, ideally, no added salt) are fine. Eat at least five portions a day. See pages 14–16 for which foods are rich in which vitamins and minerals and why you need them.

Fat

You do need some fat in your diet – but not too much – to provide body warmth and energy. There is enough for your daily needs contained naturally in foods so keep added fat to a minimum and eat it sparingly (see my Clever diet tips for losing weight on pages 26–27).

Fibre

Your body also needs fibre – it is particularly necessary for your digestive function. Eat plenty of fruit and vegetables, wholegrain cereals, and the skins on potatoes.

Liquids

You also need lots of liquid in your diet. Make sure you drink plenty of water from the tap, filtered or mineral according to your preference. If you're really not keen on water, flavour it with a low-calorie squash.

Pure fruit juices are good for you and count towards your five-a-day portions of fruit and vegetables. The vitamin C in them helps you absorb the iron in foods such as fortified breakfast cereals too. Fruit drinks do contain calories, however, so they must be counted in your daily allowance.

Tea and coffee may be drunk in moderation but preferably after or between meals, as the tannin in the beverages impairs the absorption of some essential nutrients. If you want to add milk, use skimmed or semi-skimmed. Alternatively, drink both tea and coffee black (tea with lemon is deliciously refreshing and contains hardly any calories). Don't add any sugar. If you have a sweet tooth, use artificial sweeteners, but, ideally, wean yourself off them. Learning to do without sweetness will help your new, healthy lifestyle.

Try to consume at least 300 ml/½ pt/1¼ cups of skimmed or semi-skimmed milk during the day; this includes what you put on cereal or use in cooking. If you have a lot of weight to lose, then go for the skimmed option.

Alcohol

Alcohol is not a dieter's friend. If you are trying to lose weight, it piles on 'empty' calories, so have it as a treat only. Use low-calorie mixers with spirits and go for low-strength beers. If you like wine, try having a spritzer (wine diluted with sparkling water). Whatever you do, **don't** use drink as a substitute for good, nutritious food.

Regular exercise

An active body is more likely to be a healthy body. However, one mad burst of exercise a week at the gym isn't a good idea (although it's better than nothing). You need to take more frequent, regular exercise to reap the benefit.

There are plenty of ways to exercise without jogging or work-outs. Get into the habit of walking briskly instead of wandering along. Go on foot whenever possible instead of using the car or public transport. If you take the bus, get off a stop before your usual one and walk the last part of the journey. Ride a bike if you have one. Use the stairs instead of lifts or escalators. Take up a recreational sport like tennis or swimming or join an activity like a dance class. Even gardening will burn off calories.

Bending and stretching exercises will also help to tone your muscles but seek advice before you start any exercise regime – you must do them correctly or you can cause injury. If you are going to do exercises at home, do them at a fixed time, perhaps as soon as you get out of bed or before you have your shower or bath in the morning or evening. Try to make them a regular part of your daily routine, otherwise the novelty will wear off after a few days and you won't persevere.

Vitamin and minerals in foods

I mentioned earlier that a balanced diet of fresh foods should contain sufficient vitamins and minerals to keep your body healthy, and supplements should not be necessary for the vast majority of people. However, if you have been told that you are deficient in iron, for example, you may want to increase the number of iron-rich foods in your diet. You can consult the following tables to find the foods that are particularly rich in the major vitamins and minerals.

Vitamin	Important for	Vitamin-rich foods
Vitamin A	Colour and night vision; healthy skin and mucous membranes	Liver, fortified margarines, butter, eggs, whole milk products (e.g. full-fat cheeses), green, orange and red vegetables, fish liver oils
B Vitamin complex:		
Thiamin (B_1)	Conversion of carbohydrates to energy; function of the central nervous system	Bread and other cereals, milk and milk products, potatoes, meat, yeast extract
Riboflavin (B_2)	Conversion of carbohydrates, fats and proteins to energy; healthy skin and eyes	Fortified breakfast cereals, eggs, vegetables, milk and milk products, meat (especially offal), poultry, yeast extract
Niacin (Nicotinic acid)	Conversion of carbohydrates, fats and proteins to energy	Fortified breakfast cereals, bread, potatoes, meat and meat products, poultry, fish
Vitamin B_6	Conversion of proteins, fats and carbohydrates to energy; function of the central nervous system	Potatoes and other vegetables, pulses (dried peas, beans and lentils), fruit, meat and poultry, cereals

Vitamin B$_{12}$	Function of the central nervous system; production of red blood cells; growth	Meat and meat products (especially liver), cheese, milk, eggs, fish, yeast extract, fortified breakfast cereals
Folic acid	Function of the central nervous system; production of red blood cells	Wholegrain cereals, offal, green, leafy vegetables (especially raw ones), oranges
Pantothenic acid	Conversion of fats and proteins to energy	Pulses, fortified cereals, offal, fresh vegetables, peanuts
Biotin	Conversion of fats and proteins to energy	Milk and milk products, fruit and vegetables, fish, egg yolk, cereals, offal
Vitamin C	Production of collagen for connective tissue, blood vessels and capillaries; support of the immune system and healing; absorption of iron; detoxification (for alcohol and drugs)	Potatoes, pure fruit juices, fruit, especially blackcurrants, strawberries, kiwis and citrus, vegetables, especially potatoes, green vegetables, (bell) peppers
Vitamin D	Growth and maintenance of healthy teeth and bones; absorption of calcium	Sunshine, butter, fortified margarines, fortified breakfast cereals, eggs, oily fish
Vitamin E	Protection of cell membranes; antioxidant	Wholegrain cereals, eggs, dark leafy vegetables, vegetable oils

Vitamin K	Metabolism of energy; blood clotting	Vegetables, especially brassicas (cabbage, cauliflower, etc.) and spinach
Essential fatty acids: Linoleic acid (Omega-3) Linolenic acid (Omega-6)	General good health	Oily fish, vegetable seeds and seed oils (including polyunsaturated margarines)

Mineral	Important for	Mineral-rich foods
Calcium	Healthy growth and development of bones and teeth; release of hormones in the body	Milk and milk products, canned fish (especially the bones), bread, green vegetables
Chromium	Activating insulin, which controls the use of glucose in the body	Most foods, particularly wholegrain cereals and vegetables
Copper	Production of enzymes, especially those involved with the blood and bones and the immune system; aiding neurotransmission; respiration of cells	Wholegrain cereals, vegetables, meat, oysters, nuts
Fluorine	Prevention of tooth decay	Fish, water, tea
Iodine	Regulation of many body processes, via the thyroid hormones	Meat, fish, eggs, milk and milk products, iodised salt
Iron	Formation of red blood cells; transportation and transfer of oxygen; metabolism of drugs	Potatoes and other vegetables, bread and cereal products, meat, especially offal
Magnesium	Muscle tone; enzyme activation, especially to break down proteins	Bread and cereal products, potatoes and other vegetables, milk, nuts

Manganese	Maintenance of healthy cells; activation of enzymes; helping the utilisation of calcium and potassium	Nuts, wholegrain cereals, tea
Molybdenum	Production of many enzymes, especially for the formation of uric acid; and the metabolism of DNA	Most foods, particularly vegetables and pulses
Phosphorus	Production of all cells; aiding storage of energy, membrane function, growth and reproduction	Bread and cereal products, meat and meat products, milk and milk products
Potassium	Maintenance of water levels in the body	Fruit and pure fruit juices, vegetables, milk, meat
Selenium	Production of an enzyme in red blood cells; protection of membranes	Fish, cheese, milk, eggs, meat (especially offal), cereals
Sodium and chlorine	Maintenance of water levels in the body	Bread and cereal products, meat products, milk, cooking and table salt
Zinc	Metabolism of bones; release of Vitamin A and insulin; activation of enzymes; growth; support of the immune system; taste	Milk and milk products, bread and cereal products, meat and meat products

Controlling Your Weight

Calorie counting is an efficient way of controlling your diet and so adjusting your weight. To lose weight, your energy, or calorie, intake from food and drink (that's the calories in the food you eat) needs to be less than your energy output (the number of calories you burn up through activity). Strictly speaking, the measure we refer to as 'calories' should actually be called kilocalories (units of 1,000 calories) but they are always abbreviated to kcalories, or calories.

An average man uses about 2,500 calories a day; a woman about 1,900 calories. The difference is partly because of size and partly because women tend to have a slower metabolic rate – they don't use up calories as quickly. The more active your lifestyle and the more exercise you undertake, the more calories you will use up.

If you only want to lose a small amount of weight and you want to do it fairly quickly, you should aim for a low daily calorie intake – say 1,500 calories for a man, 1,000 calories for a woman. But if you are planning a long-term, substantial weight reduction, it is much more effective to take it more slowly, aiming at, say, 1,900 calories per day for a man and 1,500 for a woman.

If you are underweight, of course, you will need to consume more calories than you burn in order to gain weight.

Your perfect weight

It is crucial that you are realistic about the weight you want to be. Having established the weight that you are aiming for, you should plan for a slow and steady weight loss, or gain, and work towards maintaining a healthy, balanced diet as your normal routine.

On page 21 is a chart, based on UK government statistics **(for adults only)**, which shows you how much you should weigh according to your height. Your bone structure will dictate whether you are at the lower end of the scale or higher up. The important thing is to be within the limits of ideal weight.

Weigh yourself first thing in the morning, preferably without clothes. If you weigh yourself when you are dressed, make sure you are wearing similar clothing each time. Check where you are on the table, then work out how much weight you need to lose or gain.

Once you've made that calculation and started your diet, weigh yourself on the same scales, in the same way, **once a week only.** Avoid the temptation to keep hopping on and off the scales, as weight fluctuates throughout the day and from day to day, which will only make you disheartened. There is usually a quick burst of weight loss in the first few days of a slimming diet, then the rate of loss will level off. Weighing yourself once a week will give you a much clearer picture of your progress. In the same way, if you are trying to put on weight, there may be an initial burst, then your weight will reach a plateau for a while before rising again.

Don't give up. If you are following a healthy and sensible balanced diet, you will be rewarded in the end.

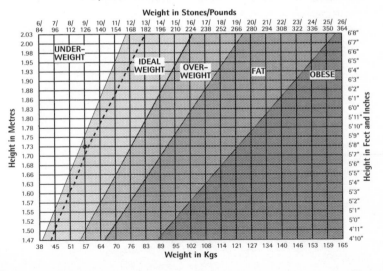

Weight in Stones/Pounds

21

Calories and exercise

Regular exercise doesn't just burn up calories, it is a vital part of a healthy lifestyle. You'll see from this list (which is based on a woman of average height and build) the difference between the number of calories you use up doing physically active tasks and the more leisurely ones.

Activity	Calories used in 30 minutes	Activity	Calories used in 30 minutes
Aerobics	210	Jogging	165
Ballroom dancing	190	Manual work, heavy	225
Climbing stairs	330	Manual work, light	120
Cycling, fast or uphill	330	Running, fast	200
Cycling, leisurely speed	120	Shopping	120
Disco dancing	205	Sleeping	30
Driving a car	60	Squash	273
Gardening, digging	240	Swimming, racing speed	300
Gardening, hoeing	105	Swimming, relaxed speed	255
Golf	195	Tennis	250
Gym work-out	210	Typing	60
Hill-walking	240	Walking, relaxed speed	120
Horse-riding, hacking	60	Walking, briskly	180
Horse-riding, trotting and cantering	180	Watching TV	45
House work	120		

Planning your diet

To keep a strict note of your calorie intake, you need to plan your day's menu, including drinks. Then look up each item and add the calorie totals together. The full amount should be equal to or less than your limit to lose weight; if you wish to gain weight, it should be above your limit. If the result is lower than your planned count for the day, you can give yourself an extra snack or another portion of healthy food, such as a vegetable or some bread with your meal. If you're over the limit and on a reducing diet, then you must find a lower-calorie alternative, perhaps grilled (broiled) fish instead of a fish pie, or fruit salad instead of apple crumble. To help you reduce your calorie count without even realising, I have included some cunning diet tips on pages 26–29.

Do read the tips for a healthy lifestyle on page 9, too. If you want your diet to work long-term and to keep fit and well, it is essential that you follow a sensible, balanced diet.

Going out for a meal

If you are trying to lose weight and you are invited out for a meal, don't panic. Most of the dishes you're likely to come across are in this book – even down to your aperitif or glass of wine. However, don't let yourself become a bore about it. Other people around you won't be dieting and if they see you constantly poring over your little guide, they will think you're obsessive. It's probably better to consult the book before you go out – you will soon get to know what are low-calorie foods and what are the blow-outs. Stick to the goodies if you can, but if you can't, don't worry. If you go over your calorie limit one day, then make sure the next day you stay under limit by a similar amount to even out your average daily intake. But be warned, this will only work if you do it on an occasional basis. You can't expect to be able to cheat all the time. It's pointless to keep going over your limit, telling yourself that tomorrow you'll be good. Try to stick to your calorie limit every day, or you won't see the benefits.

Diet and health foods

There are many ranges of special diet foods available. They are relatively expensive, however, and do not offer any guarantee that you will actually lose weight. That said, low-calorie options can be useful when you are controlling your calories.

Regulations governing food labelling mean that the word 'diet' can appear on a label only if the food is a low-calorie one. In order to be so-named, it must contain no more than 40 calories per 100 g/4 oz or 100 ml/3½ fl oz and must state clearly that it can only help weight loss if consumed as part of a calorie-controlled diet.

Many foods claim to be nutritionally 'better for you' and there are voluntary guidelines in place over what some of these definitions mean. However, they can be rather vague, and some of the products that make this claim may be no better than the standard product. The only way to be sure is to read the labels (and this book!) and see the nutritional values for yourself. Below is a guide to what the wording on the labels means.

Fat-free	Contains no more than 0.15 g of fat per 100 g.
Low in saturates	Contains no more than 3 per cent saturated fat per 100 g.
Sugar-free	Contains no more than 0.2 g sugar per 100 g.
No added sugar	Has no sugar or foods made up mainly of sugars (e.g. dried fruit or concentrated fruit juice) added to it or any of its ingredients.
Reduced-fat/ reduced-sugar	Contains at least 25 per cent less fat/sugar than the standard product.
High fibre	Contains more than 6 g fibre per 100 g.
Low-fat/ low-sugar	Contains no more than 5 g fat/sugar per 100 g.
Low-sodium	Contains no more than 40 mg sodium per 100 g.

All of the above are fairly clear. But there are other terms, commonly used on labels, that are not covered by the guidelines, and these can be more ambiguous.

Lower fat	This means the fat has less fat than the standard product, but the quantity may be reduced by only a tiny fraction!
Light or lite	This is likely to mean lower in fat but could mean lighter in weight, lighter in colour, or even lighter in texture!
Virtually fat-free	This should mean the food contains very little fat and so is a good one to look out for. But see below.
90 per cent fat-free	Sounds good – but in reality it means the product contains 10 per cent fat. This means it has more fat than one labelled 'low-fat'!

Clever diet tips for losing weight

You don't have to go on a special diet to lose weight – there are lots of ways to cut down on the calories whilst continuing to eat normal meals.

- Choose low-fat yoghurts, cheeses, cream, etc.
- Drink skimmed milk.
- Beware of cream substitutes – they often have more calories than the real thing!

- Fill up on as many vegetables or salad stuffs as you like – as long as they are not laced with gallons of oil or melted butter!
- Remove all fat or skin from meat and poultry before eating.
- Choose lean meats and trim off excess fat before cooking.
- Grill (broil) rather than fry (sauté).
- Use a low-fat spread instead of butter and add only a scraping to bread. Don't add any extra to vegetables before serving. I have given the calorie count for an **average** spreading in the book. If you can use half that amount, do so (you will reap the benefits in reduced calories!)
- Beware of spread or butter melting into hot toast and 'clumping' on new bread – you won't be able to resist adding more!
- Use only the minimum of oil for cooking and drain off any excess.
- When browning meat for a made-up dish, dry-fry rather than adding oil and spoon off any fat.
- Don't add sugar to fruits, cereals or drinks.
- Choose low-calorie brands of soft drinks, dressings, etc.
- Drink plenty of water.
- Choose fruits canned in natural juice only, not syrup, and drink unsweetened pure juices. Beware of cartons labelled as fruit juice 'drinks' – these contain sugar and other additives.

Tips to make losing weight easier

Simply reducing the quantity of food you eat will help greatly in cutting down your calorie intake. If you are normally used to very large portions, try any of the following.

- Use a smaller plate for meals.
- A glass of naturally sparkling mineral water with your meal will help fill you up. Drink it in between meals too – zip it up with a slice of lemon or lime.
- Use a strong-flavoured cheese when cooking. You won't need to add so much to give it a good flavour.
- Cut foods into smaller pieces or thinner slices and serve yourself your usual number of pieces/slices – you'll think you've had the same but you'll actually have had less.
- Keep your butter or other spread at room temperature. It will spread much more easily, so you will use much less and save lots of calories. For example, a slice of bread and butter is 169 calories, but spread thinly with warm butter it will be only 132 calories!
- Chew slowly and eat small forkfuls. Your meal will last longer, giving you time to feel more satisfied.
- Never go shopping on an empty stomach – it's too tempting.
- Try to eat meals **before** you're ravenously hungry – especially if you are going to a restaurant!

- If you go out for a meal, don't skip the starter in the hope that you'll save calories. Opt for a low-calorie one – together with the main course it will take the edge off your appetite, and with any luck you'll be able to avoid the calorie-packed desserts!
- If you feel really peckish, eat some raw carrots – or any salad vegetables, or a bunch of grapes or a few slices of apple – to keep you going and take the edge off your appetite.
- Make a drink of meat or yeast extract (such as Bovril or Marmite) – a teaspoon in a mug of boiling water. It will take the edge off your appetite and help to fill you up between meals.
- Keep a packet of sugar-free chewing gum handy and chew between meals. Alternatively, clean your teeth instead of grabbing a snack – it really works!
- Always take the trouble to make your meal look appetising. A sprinkling of parsley or vegetables attractively arranged can help you really enjoy what's on your plate rather than just eating for the sake of it.
- Don't cheat! You know if you are piling food on your plate so try to be less-than-generous. Just remember, the smaller the portion, the more you'll lose. Average portion means average, not piled high!
- Don't weigh yourself more than once a week.

How to Use This Book

Using the book is simplicity itself. You will find everything from a slice of bread to a Tournedos rossini in here, and they are all easy to find.

- All the foods are listed alphabetically so that you can find them easily without having to work out a category or recall an obscure name.
- There are clear headings and dictionary-style page headings so you can easily flick through to the place you want to find.
- All the calories given are per portion, so you don't have anything to work out. It even gives you the average calories for made-up dishes, so you don't have to weigh or calculate a thing.
- The amount of protein, carbohydrate and fat is listed for every item, plus a measure of the fibre content.
- If something may be found under two different names, I have included both and cross-referenced them.
- Prepared meals can be found under both the initial letter of the recipe title and also under the main ingredient. So Tandoori chicken may be found under both T for tandoori and C for chicken.

- Where a product has different variations, I have listed it under its generic name. So, for example, you'll find all the varieties of milk under M: 'Milk, skimmed', 'Milk, semi-skimmed' and so on.
- Where a food has different flavours, as do crisps (potato chips), for example, I have given an average calorie content for all the flavours. You can always check the specific food labels for the exact calorie count, but the difference is only one or two calories!

Portion sizes

To make the book really dieter-friendly, I have calculated the foods using **average** portions. To be sure of success with your diet, you must stick to these portion sizes. To make it clearer still – and harder for you to cheat – the table opposite explains exactly what I mean by each portion size. If you give yourself larger portions, you will suffer the consequences!

Food	Portion size given	Equivalent weight or size
Butter or other spreads	1 small knob	10 g/¼ oz/2 tsp
Cakes and pies	1 slice	⅛ of a standard pie or cake
Cereals These vary according to type (flakes, porridge, etc.) and are based on manufacturer's recommended serving size. Use a large serving spoon, not a measuring spoon.	3 heaped tablespoons 5 heaped tablespoons	50 g or 40 g 40 g or 30 g
Cheese	1 small wedge/1 good spoonful/1 small chunk	25 g/1 oz
Chocolate	1 standard bar	One size up from fun size. (The standard bars vary but are on average around 40 g.)
Drinks	1 small (beer/cider) 1 small glass 1 wine glass 1 tumbler 1 mug 1 single measure 1 double measure	300 ml/½ pt/1¼ cups 100 ml/3½ fl oz/scant ½ cup 120 ml/4 fl oz/½ cup 200 ml/7 fl oz/scant 1 cup 250 ml/8 fl oz/1 cup 25 ml/1 fl oz/1½ tbsp 50 ml/2 fl oz/3 tbsp
Fish	1 (piece of) fillet/1 steak	175 g/6 oz

Fruit and vegetables	3 heaped tablespoons	100 g/4 oz
	2 tablespoons	50 g/2 oz
	1 good handful	Approximately 25 g/1 oz (but it doesn't really matter as the calorie content is tiny!)
Ice cream	1 scoop	50 g/2 oz
Meat and poultry, roast	2 thick slices/3 medium slices/4 thin slices	100 g/4 oz
Sandwiches	1 round	2 medium slices of white bread, spread with butter, plus filling
Steaks	1 medium steak	175 g/6 oz
	1 large steak (T-bone)	350 g/12 oz
Noodles, all types	1 serving	50 g/2 oz uncooked
Nuts and dried fruit	1 small handful	15 g/½ oz
Pasta, all types	1 serving	75 g/3 oz uncooked
Rice, all types	1 serving	50 g/2 oz/¼ cup uncooked
Soup	2 ladlefuls	200 ml/7 fl oz/scant 1 cup
	1 mug	250 ml/8 fl oz/1 cup
Sauces and sundries	1 tablespoon	15 ml
	1 teaspoon	5 ml
Snacks	1 small bag	Crisps (chips): 25g Corn snacks, chocolate peanuts, etc: 50 g

Prepared dishes

For prepared dishes, whether home-made or bought ready-prepared, I have referred throughout to the measure '1 serving'. This means one standard, average-sized serving. If the dish is home-made, and the recipe is designed to serve four people, '1 serving' denotes a quarter of the whole dish. In the same way, if a cook–chill or frozen meal is labelled as serving two, '1 serving' will be half the dish. If you eat the whole lot, you must double the calories!

Remember also that recipes vary, so you must be sensible about the content of those you choose. If you know the version you are cooking has loads of extra cream in it, don't kid yourself it is a standard one! When calculating the calorific and nutritional content of each item and recipe, I have estimated the content of an **average** portion and **average** recipe.

Brand names

The information has been gathered using both UK and American data. Obviously different brands of a product do not have identical nutritional values and manufacturers change their recipes from time to time, so the figures I have used are averages and may vary slightly from the brands you buy. Always read your labels for the latest and most precise data.

A–Z of Calorie Values

The easy-to-follow page headings and clear presentation mean that you will quickly and easily find the items you are looking for.

You can make your own notes on favourite brands, recipe ideas and healthy food combinations at the end of each section.

Food	kCalories per portion	Portion size	Protein g	Carbo-hydrate g	Fat g	Fibre
Abbey crunch biscuits (cookies)	46	1 biscuit	1	7	2	low
Absinthe	55	1 single measure	trace	trace	trace	0
Ace chocolate bar	126	1 standard bar	1	16	6	low
Aduki beans, dried, soaked and boiled	123	3 heaped tablespoons	9	22	trace	high
Advocaat	68	1 single measure	1	7	2	0
Aero chocolate bar, mint	254	1 standard bar	3	28	13	0
Aero chocolate bar, orange	254	1 standard bar	3	28	13	0
Aero chocolate bar, milk	251	1 standard bar	3	26	13	0
Afelia (greek pork stew)	369	1 serving	24	12	28	low
After eight mints	32	1 mint	trace	6	1	0
Aioli	237	2 tablespoons	trace	trace	23	0
Alfalfa sprouts	7	1 good handful	trace	1	trace	high
All-bran, dry	68	25 g/1 oz/½ cup	3	11	1	high
All-bran, with semi-skimmed milk	139	5 heaped tablespoons	8	16	3	high
All-bran, with skimmed milk	123	5 heaped tablespoons	8	16	1	high
Almond biscuits (cookies)	46	1 biscuit	1	6	2	low
Almond danish pastry	420	1 pastry	6	46	24	medium
Almond macaroon	120	1 macaroon	3	13	7	medium
Almond paste	101	25 g/1 oz	1	17	4	medium
Almond slice	132	1 slice	2	21	5	low

Food	kCalories per portion	Portion size	Protein g	Carbo-hydrate g	Fat g	Fibre
Almonds, fresh, shelled	**153**	25 g/1 oz/2 tbsp	5	2	14	high
Almonds, ground	**46**	1 tablespoon	3	trace	4	high
Almonds, roasted	**95**	1 small handful	3	1	9	high
Almonds, sugared	**15**	1 sweet (candy)	trace	3	trace	high
Alpen, dry	**91**	25 g/1 oz/¼ cup	2	16	2	high
Alpen, with semi-skimmed milk	**203**	3 heaped tablespoons	8	33	5	high
Alpen, with skimmed milk	**189**	3 heaped tablespoons	8	33	3	high
Alpen, no added sugar, dry	**89**	25 g/1 oz/¼ cup	3	15	2	high
Alpen, no added sugar, with semi-skimmed milk	**200**	3 heaped tablespoons	9	31	5	high
Alpen, no added sugar, with skimmed milk	**184**	3 heaped tablespoons	9	31	3	high
Alpen nutty crunch, dry	**95**	25 g/1 oz/¼ cup	2	16	2	high
Alpen nutty crunch, with semi-skimmed milk	**209**	3 heaped tablespoons	8	32	6	high
Alpen nutty crunch, with skimmed milk	**193**	3 heaped tablespoons	8	32	4	high
Alphabetti spaghetti, canned	**135**	1 small can	4	28	1	medium
Alphabetti spaghetti, on toast	**304**	1 small can plus 1 slice of buttered toast	7	46	9	medium
Amaretti biscuits (cookies)	**21**	1 biscuit	trace	4	trace	low
Amaretto liqueur	**80**	1 single measure	0	7	0	0

Food	kCalories per portion	Portion size	Protein g	Carbo-hydrate g	Fat g	Fibre
American hard gums	**135**	1 small tube	2	40	0	0
American muffin, plain	**169**	1 muffin	5	24	6	medium
American pancake	**60**	1 pancake	2	8	2	low
Anchovies, canned	**12**	1 fillet	1	0	1	0
Anchovies, fresh, grilled (broiled)	**98**	1 fish	15	0	4	0
Anchovy essence (extract)	**7**	1 teaspoon	1	0	trace	0
Anchovy paste	**20**	1 tablespoon	3	trace	1	0
Angel cake	**77**	1 slice	1	12	trace	low
Angel delight, all flavours, made with semi-skimmed milk	**115** (average)	1 serving	3	16	4	0
Angel delight, all flavours, made with skimmed milk	**105** (average)	1 serving	3	16	2	0
Angel delight, sugar-free, all flavours, made with semi-skimmed milk	**115** (average)	1 serving	3	13	5	0
Angel delight, sugar-free, all flavours, made with skimmed milk	**105** (average)	1 serving	3	13	4	0
Angel hair (pasta strands), dried, boiled	**239**	1 serving	8	51	2	medium
Angel hair, fresh, boiled	**301**	1 serving	11	57	2	medium

Food	kCalories per portion	Portion size	Protein g	Carbo-hydrate g	Fat g	Fibre
Angels on horseback	37	1 oyster plus ½ rasher (slice) of bacon	4	trace	3	0
Anis	55	1 single measure	trace	trace	0	0
Aniseed balls	81	1 small tube	trace	87	trace	0
Antipasti, mixed	244	1 serving	24	11	13	high
Anzac biscuits (cookies)	98	1 biscuit	2	4	5	low
Apple	47	1 fruit, unpeeled	trace	12	trace	high
Apple, cooking (tart)	35	1 large fruit, peeled	trace	9	trace	medium
Apple, cooking, baked, sweetened	140	1 large fruit	1	12	trace	high
Apple, dried rings	13	1 ring	trace	3	trace	high
Apple, dried rings, stewed	66	3 heaped tablespoons	trace	13	trace	high
Apple, dried rings, stewed with sugar	106	3 heaped tablespoons	trace	17	trace	high
Apple, stewed	33	3 heaped tablespoons	trace	8	trace	medium
Apple, stewed with sugar	74	3 heaped tablespoons	trace	19	trace	medium
Apple, toffee	251	1 medium fruit	4	66	trace	high
Apple amber	340	1 serving	2	14	2	medium
Apple and blackcurrant juice drink	74	1 tumbler	trace	16	trace	0
Apple and mango juice drink	67	1 tumbler	0	0	trace	0
Apple betty	260	1 serving	2	39	10	medium
Apple cake	252	1 slice	3	32	10	medium

Food	kCalories per portion	Portion size	Protein g	Carbo-hydrate g	Fat g	Fibre
Apple charlotte	**263**	1 serving	3	41	9	medium
Apple chutney	**30**	1 tablespoon	trace	3	trace	low
Apple croissant	**144**	1 croissant	4	21	5	medium
Apple crumble	**297**	1 serving	3	51	10	medium
Apple danish pastry	**298**	1 pastry	6	51	18	medium
Apple drink, sparkling	**78**	1 tumbler	trace	19	trace	0
Apple drink, sparkling, low-calorie	**9**	1 tumbler	trace	2	trace	0
Apple dumpling	**287**	1 dumpling	3	54	8	high
Apple fritter	**136**	1 fritter	2	26	5	medium
Apple jelly (clear conserve)	**67**	1 tablespoon	0	17	0	low
Apple juice	**76**	1 tumbler	trace	10	trace	low
Apple juice drink, diluted	**88**	1 tumbler	trace	21	trace	0
Apple pie	**290**	1 slice	3	39	14	medium
Apple sauce	**25**	1 tablespoon	trace	2	trace	medium
Apple snow	**97**	1 serving	4	19	1	medium
Apple strudel	**194**	1 slice	2	29	8	medium
Apple tango	**78**	1 tumbler	trace	19	trace	0
Apple tango, light	**9**	1 tumbler	trace	2	trace	0
Apple turnover	**284**	1 turnover	4	31	16	medium
Apricot	**17**	1 fruit	trace	4	trace	medium

Food	kCalories per portion	Portion size	Protein g	Carbo- hydrate g	Fat g	Fibre
Apricot and almond danish pastry	270	1 pastry	6	38	12	medium
Apricot bites, dry	70	25 g/1 oz/½ cup	3	13	1	high
Apricot bites, with semi-skimmed milk	169	3 heaped tablespoons	9	27	2	high
Apricot bites, with skimmed milk	153	3 heaped tablespoons	9	27	3	high
Apricot brandy	56	1 single measure	trace	7	0	0
Apricot jam (conserve)	39	1 tablespoon	trace	10	0	0
Apricot juice	78	1 tumbler	1	20	trace	0
Apricot nectar	112	1 tumbler	1	32	trace	0
Apricot sorbet	57	1 scoop	trace	19	trace	low
Apricots, canned in natural juice	34	3 heaped tablespoons	trace	8	trace	medium
Apricots, canned in syrup	63	3 heaped tablespoons	trace	16	trace	medium
Apricots, dried	15	1 fruit	trace	3	trace	high
Apricots, dried, stewed	85	3 heaped tablespoons	1	22	trace	high
Apricots, dried, stewed with sugar	113	3 heaped tablespoons	1	29	trace	high
Apricots, stewed	31	3 heaped tablespoons	1	7	trace	medium
Apricots, stewed with sugar	61	3 heaped tablespoons	1	15	trace	medium
Arbroath smokies, grilled (broiled), with butter	239	1 fish	37	0	10	0

Food	kCalories per portion	Portion size	Protein g	Carbo- hydrate g	Fat g	Fibre
Archers peach liqueur	65	1 single measure	trace	8	0	0
Arctic roll	100	1 slice	2	16	3	low
Arrowroot biscuits (cookies), thin	35	1 biscuit	1	7	2	low
Artichoke, globe, boiled	70	1 artichoke	0	3	0	medium
Artichoke, with melted butter	181	1 artichoke	1	3	13	medium
Artichoke hearts, canned, drained	8	1 heart	1	1	trace	medium
Artichoke vinaigrette	211	1 artichoke	1	3	22	medium
Artichokes, Jerusalem, boiled	41	3 heaped tablespoons	2	11	0	high
Asparagus, canned, drained	24	½ medium can	3	1	trace	medium
Asparagus, roasted in olive oil	161	6 thick or 10 thin spears	3	1	16	medium
Asparagus, steamed or boiled	26	6 thick or 10 thin spears	3	2	2	medium
Asparagus, with melted butter	137	6 thick or 10 thin spears	3	1	13	medium
Asparagus quiche	320	1 slice	13	18	22	medium
Asparagus soup, cream of, canned	132	2 ladlefuls	2	10	10	low
Asparagus soup, cream of, instant	143	1 mug	1	20	6	low
Asparagus soup, home-made	167	2 ladlefuls	3	7	14	high

Food	kCalories per portion	Portion size	Protein g	Carbo-hydrate g	Fat g	Fibre
Aubergine (eggplant), fried (sautéed) in oil	302	¼ aubergine	1	3	32	medium
Aubergine, steamed or boiled	28	¼ aubergine	1	3	trace	medium
Aubergine, stuffed with meat	510	½ aubergine	46	28	24	medium
Aubergine, stuffed with savoury rice	523	½ aubergine	8	26	14	high
Aubergine dip	20	2 tablespoons	1	4	1	medium
Austrian coffee cake	488	1 slice	5	41	32	low
Austrian smoked cheese	60	¼ barrel (25 g/1 oz)	4	trace	3	0
Avgolemono soup	74	2 ladlefuls	3	5	2	low
Avocado	286	1 medium fruit	3	3	29	medium
Avocado, baked, with tomato and cheese	196	½ avocado	5	4	18	medium
Avocado, with prawns (shrimp) in cocktail sauce	356	½ avocado	13	2	32	medium
Avocado vinaigrette	240	½ avocado	1	1	25	medium

Food	kCalories per portion	Portion size	Protein g	Carbo-hydrate g	Fat g	Fibre
Babybel cheese	53	1 cheese	4	0	4	0
Bacardi	50	1 single measure	trace	trace	trace	0
Bacardi and coke	94	1 single measure plus 1 mixer	trace	6	0	0
Bacardi and diet coke	56	1 single measure plus 1 mixer	trace	trace	0	0
Baclava	322	1 pastry	5	40	17	medium
Bacon, back, lean, fried (sautéed)	133	1 rasher (slice)	13	0	16	0
Bacon, back, lean, grilled (broiled)	117	1 rasher	12	0	8	0
Bacon, joint, boiled	325	2 medium slices	20	0	27	0
Bacon, joint, honey-roasted	346	2 medium slices	20	4	27	0
Bacon, streaky, fried	149	1 rasher	7	0	13	0
Bacon, streaky, grilled	127	1 rasher	7	0	11	0
Bacon and egg quiche	387	1 slice	15	17	31	low
Bacon and egg mcmuffin	346	1 muffin	20	26	18	medium
Bacon and mushroom pizza, deep-pan	340	1 slice	10	35	16	medium
Bacon and mushroom pizza, thin-crust	290	1 slice	10	25	15	medium
Bacon cheeseburger	400	1 burger	24	27	22	low
Bacon sandwiches	538	1 round	30	34	32	medium

Food	kCalories per portion	Portion size	Protein g	Carbohydrate g	Fat g	Fibre
Bagel	**228**	1 bagel	7	44	3	medium
Bagna cauda	**499**	1 individual pot	6	0	52	0
Baguette	**364**	1 small	11	75	2	medium
Bailey's irish cream	**80**	1 single measure	trace	6	4	0
Baked alaska	**339**	1 serving	8	62	8	low
Baked beans	**168**	1 small can	10	31	1	high
Baked beans, barbecued	**164**	1 small can	10	30	1	high
Baked beans, on toast	**323**	1 small can plus 1 slice of toast	14	49	10	high
Baked beans, reduced-sugar and reduced-salt	**146**	1 small can	11	25	1	high
Baked beans, reduced-sugar and reduced-salt, on toast	**301**	1 small can plus 1 slice of toast	14	43	10	high
Baked beans, with bacon	**182**	1 small can plus 2 rashers (slices) of bacon	12	26	3	high
Baked beans, with burgers, canned	**206**	1 small can	13	26	6	high
Baked beans, with sausages, canned	**220**	1 small can	10	26	9	high
Baked beans, with vegetarian sausages, canned	**240**	1 small can	11	63	trace	high
Bakewell slice	**156**	1 slice	1	22	7	medium
Bakewell tart	**297**	1 slice	4	37	15	medium

Food	kCalories per portion	Portion size	Protein g	Carbo-hydrate g	Fat g	Fibre
Balsamic vinegar	1	1 tablespoon	trace	trace	0	0
Bamboo shoots	6	2 tablespoons	1	trace	trace	medium
Banana	95	1 medium fruit	1	23	trace	medium
Banana, dried slices	78	1 small handful	trace	9	5	medium
Banana bread	246	1 slice	2	45	7	medium
Banana custard	50	5 tablespoons	1	8	1	0
Banana flambé	250	1 banana	1	28	8	medium
Banana fritter	175	1 fritter	3	33	5	medium
Banana milkshake, fresh, made with semi-skimmed milk	163	1 tumbler	6	31	3	medium
Banana milkshake, fresh, made with skimmed milk	144	1 tumbler	6	31	trace	medium
Banana sandwiches	399	1 round	7	57	17	medium
Banana split	481	1 serving	10	77	16	medium
Bananabix, dry	92	25 g/1 oz/½ cup	2	18	trace	high
Bananabix, with semi-skimmed milk	207	3 heaped tablespoons	8	35	4	high
Bananabix, with skimmed milk	191	3 heaped tablespoons	8	35	3	high
Bangers and mash	462	2 sausages plus 4 spoonfuls of mash	17	43	20	medium
Banoffee pie	574	1 slice	10	68	23	medium

Food	kCalories per portion	Portion size	Protein g	Carbo-hydrate g	Fat g	Fibre
Barbecue sauce	11	1 tablespoon	trace	1	trace	0
Barbecued baked beans	164	1 small can	10	30	1	high
Barbecued chicken	287	1 chicken portion	46	1	10	0
Barbecued pork chop	210	1 chop	28	1	9	0
Barbecued spare ribs	288	2 ribs	25	2	16	0
Barley sugar	96	1 stick	trace	24	0	0
Barley water, all flavours	40 (average)	1 tumbler	trace	9	trace	0
Barley water, all flavours, no added sugar	6 (average)	1 tumbler	trace	1	trace	0
Barley wine	120	1 small bottle	1	11	trace	0
Bass, fried (sautéed), in seasoned flour	261	1 piece of fillet	32	5	12	low
Bass, grilled (broiled)	142	1 piece of fillet	31	0	2	0
Bass, poached	141	1 piece of fillet	32	0	2	0
Bass, stuffed, baked	182	1 serving	32	1	4	low
Bath bun	263	1 bun	8	45	15	medium
Bath olivers	50	1 biscuit (cookie)	1	8	2	low
Battenburg cake	370	1 slice	6	50	17	medium
Bavarian smoked cheese	60	¼ barrel (25 g/1 oz)	4	trace	3	0
Bavarois, all flavours	308 (average)	1 serving	7	17	23	0
Bean and cheese enchiladas	547	2 enchiladas	28	82	14	high

Food	kCalories per portion	Portion size	Protein g	Carbohydrate g	Fat g	Fibre
Bean salad	120	3 heaped tablespoons	4	12	5	high
Beanburger, spicy	112	1 burger	9	4	6	medium
Beans *See individual varieties, e.g. Runner beans*						
Beansprouts	8	1 good handful	1	1	trace	high
Béarnaise sauce	275	5 tablespoons	3	7	27	low
Béchamel sauce, made with semi-skimmed milk	96	5 tablespoons	3	8	6	low
Beef, boiled	326	2 thick slices	28	0	24	0
Beef, corned	54	1 slice	7	0	3	0
Beef, grillsteak, grilled (broiled)	185	1 steak	11	8	12	low
Beef, minced (ground), in gravy, canned	230	½ large can	19	14	11	0
Beef, minced, lean, stewed	229	1 serving	23	0	15	0
Beef, roast, lean	225	3 thin slices	28	0	19	0
Beef, steak *See Steak*						
Beef, stewed in gravy	335	1 serving	47	0	16	0
Beef, stewed in gravy, canned	254	½ large can	32	8	10	0
Beef and cheese enchiladas	644	2 enchiladas	24	60	36	low
Beef and tomato soup, canned	88	2 ladlefuls	5	10	2	low
Beef and tomato soup, instant	72	1 mug	1	15	1	0

Food	kCalories per portion	Portion size	Protein g	Carbo-hydrate g	Fat g	Fibre
Beef and vegetable stir-fry	433	1 serving	26	71	5	high
Beef broth, canned	76	2 ladlefuls	4	13	1	medium
Beef carbonnade (in beer)	384	1 serving	30	15	21	low
Beef casserole	360	1 serving	28	13	21	medium
Beef chop suey	297	1 serving	23	34	6	medium
Beef chow mein	408	1 serving	19	43	18	high
Beef consommé, canned	14	2 ladlefuls	3	1	trace	0
Beef consommé, jellied	21	2 ladlefuls	4	1	trace	0
Beef curry, home-made	905	1 serving	37	10	77	medium
Beef curry, home-made, with rice	1153	1 serving	42	66	79	medium
Beef curry, retail	411	1 serving	40	19	18	medium
Beef curry, retail, with rice	657	1 serving	43	82	19	medium
Beef fajitas	528	2 fajitas	40	79	8	medium
Beef goulash	406	1 serving	28	16	22	medium
Beef in oyster sauce	204	1 serving	24	10	8	low
Beef kheema	826	1 serving	36	1	75	low
Beef koftas	441	1 serving	28	4	35	low
Beef olives	494	2 olives	58	20	18	low
Beef pie	460	1 individual pie	18	32	28	low
Beef pot roast, with vegetables	420	1 serving	44	14	15	medium

Food	kCalories per portion	Portion size	Protein g	Carbohydrate g	Fat g	Fibre
Beef risotto	452	1 serving	16	54	29	low
Beef satay	222	1 skewer	25	6	11	low
Beef sausages, thick, fried (sautéed)	108	1 sausage	5	6	7	low
Beef sausages, thick, grilled (broiled)	106	1 sausage	5	6	7	low
Beef sausages, thin, fried	54	1 sausage	3	4	4	low
Beef sausages, thin, grilled	53	1 sausage	3	4	4	low
Beef spread	35	1 tablespoon	1	2	3	low
Beef steak pudding	684	1 serving	33	57	37	medium
Beef stew	360	1 serving	28	13	21	medium
Beef stroganoff	361	1 serving	22	8	25	medium
Beef teriyaki	128	1 serving	18	2	4	low
Beef wellington	527	1 serving	37	23	33	low
Beef with mushrooms, chinese	320	1 serving	37	44	6	low
Beef with pineapple, chinese	337	1 serving	23	47	6	low
See also Boeuf						
Beefburger, fried (sautéed)	125	1 burger	6	trace	11	0
Beefburger, grilled (broiled)	122	1 burger	6	trace	11	0
Beefburger, in a bun, quarterpounder	321	1 burger in a bun	22	27	15	medium
Beefburger, in a bun, small	246	1 burger in a bun	11	23	13	medium

Food	kCalories per portion	Portion size	Protein g	Carbo-hydrate g	Fat g	Fibre
Beer, bitter	**96**	1 small	1	7	trace	0
Beer, extra-strength	**216**	1 small	2	18	trace	0
Beer, pale ale	**96**	1 small	1	6	trace	0
Beerwurst	**55**	1 slice	3	trace	4	0
Beetroot (red beet)	**36**	1 medium	2	7	trace	medium
Beetroot, boiled	**46**	1 medium	2	9	trace	medium
Beetroot, pickled	**28**	5 slices	1	6	trace	medium
Bel paese cheese	**87**	1 small wedge	5	trace	7	0
Belgian bun	**192**	1 bun	5	30	5	low
Belgian endive See Chicory						
Belgian ham, dry-cured	**21**	1 slice	4	0	1	0
Bell pepper See Pepper						
Benedictine	**90**	1 single measure	0	6	0	0
Big bar ace	**204**	1 standard bar	2	25	10	low
Big breakfast	**591**	1 meal	26	40	36	high
Big fish sandwich	**720**	1 bun	23	59	43	high
Big mac	**493**	1 burger	27	44	23	high
Bigarde sauce	**123**	5 tablespoons	5	10	4	low
Biscotti	**39**	1 biscuit (cookie)	1	6	1	low
Biscuits (cookies), chocolate, full-coated	**131**	1 biscuit	1	17	7	low

Food	kCalories per portion	Portion size	Protein g	Carbo-hydrate g	Fat g	Fibre
Biscuits, chocolate, half-coated	84	1 biscuit	1	11	4	low
Biscuits, cream-filled	77	1 biscuit	1	10	4	low
Biscuits, semi-sweet	46	1 biscuit	1	7	2	low
Biscuits, short, sweet	47	1 biscuit	1	6	2	low
Biscuits, wafer, cream-filled	39	1 biscuit	trace	5	3	low
See also individual names, e.g. Hobnob						
Bitter lemon, sparkling	68	1 tumbler	trace	16	0	0
Bitter orange, sparkling	68	1 tumbler	trace	16	0	0
Black bean sauce	22	1 tablespoon	1	3	trace	0
Black beans, dried, soaked and cooked	103	3 heaped tablespoons	trace	18	trace	high
Black cherries, canned in syrup	71	3 heaped tablespoons	0	0	trace	low
Black cherry cheesecake	242	1 slice	6	33	11	low
Black cherry jam (conserve)	39	1 tablespoon	trace	10	0	0
Black cherry jam, reduced-sugar	6	1 tablespoon	trace	5	0	0
Black forest gateau	432	1 slice	7	65	18	low
Black forest ham	29	1 thin slice	4	trace	2	0
Black gram, boiled	45	1 serving	4	7	trace	low

Food	kCalories per portion	Portion size	Protein g	Carbo-hydrate g	Fat g	Fibre
Black jack chew sweets (candies)	15	1 sweet	0	3	trace	0
Black pudding, fried (sautéed)	305	2 thick slices	13	15	22	low
Black velvet	168	1 cocktail	1	5	0	0
Blackberries	25	3 heaped tablespoons	1	5	trace	high
Blackberries, stewed	21	3 heaped tablespoons	1	4	trace	medium
Blackberries, stewed with sugar	56	3 heaped tablespoons	1	14	trace	medium
Blackberry and apple crumble	297	1 serving	3	51	10	medium
Blackberry and apple pie	281	1 slice	3	11	39	medium
Blackberry jam (conserve)	39	1 tablespoon	trace	10	0	0
Blackcurrant and apple pie	378	1 slice	3	56	16	medium
Blackcurrant and apple squash, diluted	58	1 tumbler	0	15	0	0
Blackcurrant cheesecake	260	1 slice	3	38	12	low
Blackcurrant cordial, diluted	103	1 tumbler	trace	27	0	0
Blackcurrant crumble	298	1 serving	3	51	10	medium
Blackcurrant jam (conserve)	39	1 tablespoon	trace	10	0	0
Blackcurrant jam, reduced-sugar	6	1 tablespoon	trace	5	0	0
Blackcurrant juice drink	120	1 tumbler	trace	32	trace	0
Blackcurrant pastilles	131	1 small tube	3	32	0	0

Food	kCalories per portion	Portion size	Protein g	Carbo- hydrate g	Fat g	Fibre
Blackcurrant pie	**282**	1 slice	3	34	13	medium
Blackcurrant sorbet	**65**	1 scoop	trace	17	trace	0
Blackcurrants	**28**	4 tablespoons	1	7	trace	high
Blackcurrants, canned in natural juice	**31**	3 heaped tablespoons	1	8	trace	medium
Blackcurrants, canned in syrup	**72**	3 heaped tablespoons	1	18	trace	medium
Blackcurrants, stewed with sugar	**58**	3 heaped tablespoons	1	15	trace	medium
Black-eyed beans, dried, soaked and cooked	**116**	3 heaped tablespoons	9	20	1	high
Blancmange	**165**	1 serving	5	23	6	low
Blewits, fried (sautéed)	**78**	2 tablespoons	1	trace	8	low
Blewits, stewed	**6**	2 tablespoons	1	trace	trace	low
Blinis	**60**	1 pancake	2	8	2	low
Blintzes	**86**	1 pancake	8	11	1	low
Bloater, grilled (broiled)	**298**	1 fish	31	0	19	0
Bloater paste	**5**	1 teaspoon	trace	1	trace	low
Bloody mary	**69**	1 cocktail	1	3	trace	low
Bloomer loaf	**70**	1 medium slice	3	15	1	low
BLT	**650**	1 round	30	34	35	medium
Blue brie cheese	**106**	1 small wedge	4	trace	10	0
Blue chartreuse	**78**	1 single measure	trace	7	0	0
Blue cheese dip	**145**	1 small pot	1	trace	12	0

Food	kCalories per portion	Portion size	Protein g	Carbo-hydrate g	Fat g	Fibre
Blue cheese dressing	77	1 tablespoon	1	1	8	0
Blue cheese dressing, low-calorie	16	1 tablespoon	trace	2	1	0
Blue riband chocolate wafer	108	1 standard bar	1	13	6	low
Blue stilton cheese	103	1 small wedge	6	trace	9	0
Blueberries	56	3 heaped tablespoons	1	14	trace	medium
Blueberries, canned in syrup	88	3 heaped tablespoons	1	22	trace	medium
Blueberries, dried	44	1 small handful	trace	12	trace	high
Blueberries, stewed	51	3 heaped tablespoons	trace	12	trace	medium
Blueberries, stewed with sugar	81	3 heaped tablespoons	trace	22	trace	medium
Blueberry buster muffin	408	1 muffin	4	47	21	medium
Blueberry muffin	294	1 large muffin	5	38	14	medium
Blueberry pie	290	1 slice	3	39	14	medium
Bluefish, grilled (broiled)	186	1 fillet	30	0	6	0
Boasters biscuits (cookies), all flavours	90 (average)	1 biscuit	1	20	5	low
Bockwurst	199	1 sausage	9	trace	18	0
Boeuf bourguignon	450	1 serving	31	7	33	low
Boeuf en daube	351	1 serving	39	14	13	medium
See also Beef						
Boiled beef with carrots and dumplings	474	1 serving	36	29	26	medium
Boiled sweets (candies)	15	1 sweet	trace	5	trace	0

Food	kCalories per portion	Portion size	Protein g	Carbo-hydrate g	Fat g	Fibre
Bologna sausage	57	1 slice	3	trace	5	0
Bolognese sauce	217	5 tablespoons	12	5	17	low
Bolony sausage	57	1 slice	3	trace	5	0
Bombay mix snack	75	1 small handful	1	2	5	high
Bon bel cheese	78	1 small wedge	6	0	6	0
Bon-bons	28	1 sweet (candy)	0	6	trace	0
Bonito, grilled (broiled)	195	1 piece of fillet	34	0	7	0
Boost chocolate bar	295	1 standard bar	3	34	16	low
Bordelaise sauce	133	5 tablespoons	5	2	4	0
Borlotti beans, canned, drained	112	3 heaped tablespoons	5	8	trace	high
Borlotti beans, dried, soaked and cooked	116	3 heaped tablespoons	6	18	1	high
Bortsch	25	2 ladlefuls	3	1	1	high
Bortsch, jellied	50	2 ladlefuls	9	1	1	high
Boston baked beans	133	1 serving	7	26	1	high
Boudoir biscuits (lady fingers)	40	1 finger	1	6	1	low
Bouillabaisse	159	2 ladlefuls	16	21	2	medium
Bouillabaise with rouille	310	2 ladlefuls	17	23	17	medium
Bounty bar, milk chocolate	289	1 standard bar	3	32	15	low
Bounty bar, plain (semi-sweet) chocolate	276	1 standard bar	2	33	15	low
Bounty, ice cream bar	299	1 standard bar	4	24	21	low

Food	kCalories per portion	Portion size	Protein g	Carbo-hydrate g	Fat g	Fibre
Bourbon	60	1 single measure	trace	trace	0	0
Bourbon biscuits (cookies)	63	1 biscuit	1	9	3	low
Bournville chocolate	250	1 standard bar	2	30	13	0
Bournvita, made with semi-skimmed milk	145	1 mug	9	19	4	low
Bournvita, made with skimmed milk	137	1 mug	9	20	2	low
Boursin cheese, all flavours	77 (average)	1 good tablespoon	2	1	7	0
Boursin, light, all flavours	28 (average)	1 good tablespoon	2	1	2	0
Bovril	3	1 teaspoon	2	trace	trace	0
Bran, oat	51	1 tablespoon	2	9	1	high
Bran, wheat	31	1 tablespoon	2	4	1	high
Bran muffin	163	1 muffin	4	24	6	high
Brandy	55	1 single measure	trace	trace	0	0
Brandy alexander	270	1 cocktail	trace	6	18	0
Brandy butter	73	1 tablespoon	trace	8	4	0
Brandy sauce, made with semi-skimmed milk	50	5 tablespoons	1	5	2	low
Brandy sauce, made with skimmed milk	47	5 tablespoons	1	5	trace	low
Brandy snaps	57	1 snap	trace	10	2	low

Food	kCalories per portion	Portion size	Protein g	Carbo-hydrate g	Fat g	Fibre
Brandy sour	57	1 cocktail	trace	trace	trace	0
Branflakes, dry	80	25 g/1 oz/½ cup	2	16	1	high
Branflakes, with semi skimmed milk	185	5 heaped tablespoons	8	33	3	high
Branflakes, with skimmed milk	169	5 heaped tablespoons	8	33	1	high
Branflakes, with sultanas (golden raisins), dry	80	25 g/1 oz/½ cup	2	16	trace	high
Branflakes, with sultanas, with skimmed milk	169	5 heaped tablespoons	8	33	1	high
Branflakes, with sultanas, with semi-skimmed milk	185	5 heaped tablespoons	8	33	3	high
Bratwurst, fried (sautéed)	256	1 sausage	12	2	22	0
Brazil nut, shelled	23	1 nut	1	trace	3	high
Brazil nut toffee	39.3	1 toffee	trace	5	2	low
Brazils, chocolate	49	1 sweet (candy)	1	3	4	high
Bread, brown, medium-sliced	78	1 slice	3	16	1	medium
Bread, brown, medium-sliced, toasted	80	1 slice	3	16	1	medium
Bread, brown, thick-sliced	109	1 slice	4	22	1	medium
Bread, brown, thin-sliced	65	1 slice	2	13	1	medium
Bread, granary, medium-sliced	94	1 slice	4	18	1	medium
Bread, granary, medium-sliced, toasted	96	1 slice	4	18	1	medium

Food	kCalories per portion	Portion size	Protein g	Carbo-hydrate g	Fat g	Fibre
Bread, granary, thick-sliced	117	1 slice	5	23	2	medium
Bread, softgrain medium-sliced,	76	1 slice	3	15	1	medium
Bread, softgrain, medium-sliced, toasted	85	1 slice	3	18	1	medium
Bread, softgrain, thick-sliced	106	1 slice	5	21	1	medium
Bread, white, medium-sliced	78	1 slice	3	17	trace	low
Bread, white, medium-sliced, toasted	81	1 slice	3	18	trace	low
Bread, white, thick-sliced	108	1 slice	4	23	trace	low
Bread, white, thin-sliced	65	1 slice	2	14	trace	low
Bread, wholemeal, medium-sliced	77	1 slice	3	15	1	high
Bread, wholemeal, medium-sliced, toasted	79	1 slice	3	15	1	high
Bread, wholemeal, thick-sliced	107	1 slice	5	21	1	high
Bread, wholemeal, thin-sliced	64	1 slice	3	12	1	high
Bread, with butter	152 (average)	1 medium slice	3	17	9	low
Bread, with low-fat spread	117 (average)	1 medium slice	3	17	4	low
Bread pudding	297	1 serving	6	50	10	medium
Bread and butter pudding	280	1 serving	10	31	13	low
Bread roll, baton	182	1 roll	6	38	1	medium

Food	kCalories per portion	Portion size	Protein g	Carbo-hydrate g	Fat g	Fibre
Bread roll, brown	134	1 roll	5	26	2	medium
Bread roll, crusty	140	1 roll	5	29	2	low
Bread roll, finger	107	1 roll	4	21	2	low
Bread roll, granary	117	1 roll	5	23	1	medium
Bread roll, hamburger bun	132	1 bun	4	24	2	low
Bread roll, soft white bap	134	1 roll	5	26	2	low
Bread roll, starch-reduced	50	1 roll	2	10	trace	low
Bread roll, wholemeal	120	1 roll	4	24	1	high
Bread roll, with butter	214 (average)	1 roll	13	29	9	low
Bread roll, with low-fat spread	179 (average)	1 roll	14	29	5	low
Bread sauce, made with semi-skimmed milk	**14**	1 tablespoon	1	2	trace	low
Bread sauce, made with skimmed milk	12	1 tablespoon	1	2	trace	low
Breadfruit	**396**	1 medium fruit	4	104	trace	high
Breadfruit, canned, drained	66	3 heaped tablespoons	1	16	trace	medium
Breadsticks	**20**	1 stick	1	3	trace	low
Breakaway chocolate bar, caramac	**125**	1 standard bar	1	13	7	low
Breakaway, milk	114	1 standard bar	1	14	6	low
Breakfast compôte, canned	**73**	3 heaped tablespoons	trace	17	trace	high

Food	kCalories per portion	Portion size	Protein g	Carbohydrate g	Fat g	Fibre
Bream, fried (sautéed) in seasoned flour	261	1 piece of fillet	32	5	12	low
Bream, grilled (broiled)	142	1 piece of fillet	31	0	2	0
Bream, poached	141	1 piece of fillet	32	0	2	0
Bresaola	15	1 thin slice	3	trace	trace	0
Bresse bleu cheese	106	1 small wedge	4	trace	10	0
Brie cheese	80	1 small wedge	5	trace	7	0
Brill, fried (sautéed) in egg and breadcrumbs	342	1 piece of fillet	27	13	20	low
Brill, grilled (broiled)	126	1 piece of fillet	23	0	3	0
Brill, poached	125	1 piece of fillet	25	0	2	0
Brioche	140	1 brioche	4	22	4	low
Brisket of beef, boiled	326	2 thick slices	28	0	24	0
Broad (fava) beans, boiled	48	3 heaped tablespoons	5	6	1	high
Broad beans, canned, drained	77	3 heaped tablespoons	6	13	trace	high
Broad beans, frozen, cooked	81	3 heaped tablespoons	8	12	1	high
Broccoli, steamed or boiled	33	4 medium florets	4	2	1	medium
Broccoli and cauliflower soup, instant	59	1 mug	1	8	2	low
Broccoli and cauliflower soup, packet	110	2 ladlefuls	2	15	5	medium
Broccoli and cheese quiche	320	1 slice	13	18	22	low

Food	kCalories per portion	Portion size	Protein g	Carbohydrate g	Fat g	Fibre
Broccoli and cheese soup, canned	132	2 ladlefuls	4	9	7	medium
Broccoli and cheese soup, home-made	169	2 ladlefuls	9	21	6	high
Broccoli in cheese sauce, made with semi-skimmed milk	78	1 serving	4	3	2	medium
Broccoli in cheese sauce, made with skimmed milk	65	1 serving	4	3	trace	medium
Broccoli soup	118	2 ladlefuls	6	21	2	high
Brown ale	84	1 small	1	9	trace	0
Brown betty	260	1 serving	2	39	10	medium
Brown sauce	15	1 tablespoon	trace	4	0	low
Brownie, chocolate	368	1 brownie	5	63	11	medium
Brunswick stew	444	1 serving	39	46	12	high
Brussels sprouts, steamed or boiled	35	1 serving	3	3	1	high
Brussels sprouts, with chestnuts	176	3 heaped tablespoons	2	20	43	high
Bubble and squeak	240	1 serving	3	7	18	high
Bucatini (long macaroni), dried, boiled	239	1 serving	8	51	2	medium
Bucatini, fresh, boiled	301	1 serving	11	57	2	medium
Buck rarebit	312	1 slice	17	22	19	low

Food	kCalories per portion	Portion size	Protein g	Carbo-hydrate g	Fat g	Fibre
Buckling, smoked	**520**	1 fish	26	0	44	0
Buckwheat noodles, boiled	**228**	1 serving	11	48	trace	low
Buckwheat pancakes	**45**	1 pancake	2	6	2	low
Bulgar (cracked wheat), cooked	**177**	3 heaped tablespoons	6	29	4	medium
Buns See *individual flavours, e.g.* Currant bun						
Burger bun	**132**	1 bun	4	24	2	low
Burgers See *individual varieties, e.g.* Hamburger						
Burritos, with beans and cheese	**377**	2 burritos	15	55	12	medium
Burritos, with beef, beans and cheese	**331**	2 burritos	15	40	13	medium
Butter	**184**	25 g/1 oz/2 tbsp	trace	trace	20	0
Butter	**74**	1 small knob	trace	trace	8	0
Butter (lima) beans, canned, drained	**77**	3 heaped tablespoons	6	13	trace	high
Butter beans, dried, soaked and cooked	**103**	3 heaped tablespoons	7	18	1	high
Butter pecan ice cream	**91**	1 scoop	2	12	4	low
Butter puffs	**54**	1 biscuit	1	6	3	low
Butter sauce	**112**	5 tablespoons	3	8	8	low

Food	kCalories per portion	Portion size	Protein g	Carbo-hydrate g	Fat g	Fibre
Butter shortcake biscuits (cookies)	**50**	1 biscuit	1	7	2	low
Butter/vegetable fat spread	**165**	25 g/1 oz/2 tbsp	trace	trace	18	0
Butter/vegetable fat spread	66	1 small knob	trace	trace	7	0
Buttercream icing (frosting)	40	1 tablespoon	trace	9	3	0
Butterfly cakes	**245**	1 individual cake	2	26	15	low
Butterfly prawns (jumbo shrimp), fried (sautéed), in breadcrumbs	**405**	6 prawns	16	35	23	low
Buttermilk	**60**	150 ml/¼ pt/⅔ cup	6	8	trace	0
Butternut squash, steamed or boiled	**9**	½ medium squash	trace	2	trace	low
Butterscotch	**24**	1 piece	trace	5	trace	0
Butterscotch sauce	**145**	2 tablespoons	1	32	2	low
Butterscotch tart	**531**	1 slice	10	57	23	low

Food	kCalories per portion	Portion size	Protein g	Carbo-hydrate g	Fat g	Fibre
Cabbage, green, steamed or boiled	16	3 heaped tablespoons	1	2	trace	medium
Cabbage, red/white, pickled	3	1 tablespoon	trace	trace	0	medium
Cabbage, red/white, raw	27	3 heaped tablespoons	1	5	trace	medium
Cabbage leaves, stuffed	221	2 leaves	18	19	9	high
Cabinet pudding	233	1 serving	3	36	2	medium
Caerphilly cheese	94	1 small wedge	6	trace	8	0
Caesar salad	207	1 serving	17	6	13	medium
Café noir biscuits (cookies)	39	1 biscuit	trace	8	trace	low
Caffè latte	133	1 medium cup	6	10	8	0
Cajun chicken	366	1 serving	40	33	9	medium
Cake, chocolate	384	1 slice	5	58	14	low
Cake, light fruit	354	1 slice	5	58	13	medium
Cake, plain	393	1 slice	5	58	17	low
Cake, rich fruit	341	1 slice	4	60	11	medium
See also Sponge cake and individual flavours, e.g. Coffee cake						
Calabrese, steamed or boiled	33	4 medium florets	4	2	1	medium
Calamari rings, fried (sautéed), in batter	235	1 serving	14	19	12	low
Calippo ice lolly, any flavour	105	1 lolly	trace	26	trace	0
Calvados	55	1 single measure	trace	trace	0	0

Food	kCalories per portion	Portion size	Protein g	Carbo-hydrate g	Fat g	Fibre
Calves' liver, braised	**165**	3 thin slices	22	3	7	low
Calves' liver, fried (sautéed), in seasoned flour	**254**	3 thin slices	27	7	13	0
Calypso coffee	**218**	1 wine glass	1	7	14	0
Calzone	**470**	1 serving	18	50	24	medium
Cambozola cheese	**106**	1 small wedge	4	trace	10	0
Camembert cheese	**74**	1 small wedge	5	trace	6	0
Camp coffee, made with semi-skimmed milk	**125**	1 mug	8	15	4	0
Camp coffee, made with skimmed milk	**93**	1 mug	8	15	trace	0
Candied fruits See Glacé fruits						
Candied peel See Mixed peel						
Candy See *individual varieties*, e.g. Chocolate brazils, Lemon drops						
Candy floss	**100**	1 stick	trace	26	0	0
Cannellini beans, canned, drained	**101**	3 heaped tablespoons	8	22	1	high
Cannellini beans, dried, soaked and cooked	**103**	3 heaped tablespoons	8	17	trace	high
Cannelloni, filled with meat	**298**	2 tubes	12	24	17	medium
Cannelloni, filled with spinach and ricotta	**250**	2 tubes	9	17	16	medium

Food	kCalories per portion	Portion size	Protein g	Carbo-hydrate g	Fat g	Fibre
Cantal cheese	101	1 small wedge	6	trace	8	0
Canteloupe melon	57	½ melon	2	13	trace	medium
Cape gooseberries	3	1 fruit	trace	trace	trace	low
Cappellini (pasta strands), dried, boiled	239	1 serving	8	51	2	medium
Cappellini, fresh, boiled	301	1 serving	11	57	2	medium
Caper sauce, made with semi-skimmed milk	103	5 tablespoons	4	10	6	low
Caper sauce, made with skimmed milk	93	5 tablespoons	4	10	5	low
Capercaillie, roast	173	¼ bird	31	0	5	0
Capers, pickled	7	1 tablespoon	trace	2	0	low
Capon, roast, with skin	216	3 medium slices	23	0	14	0
Capon, roast, without skin	148	3 medium slices	25	0	5	0
Caponata	85	1 slice	3	15	1	medium
Cappelletti (stuffed pasta), dried, all stuffings	291 (average)	1 serving	9	45	6	medium
Cappelletti, fresh, all stuffings	229 (average)	1 serving	9	40	4	medium
Cappuccino	101	1 medium cup	2	7	6	0
Capsicum See Pepper						
Caramac chocolate bar	170	1 standard bar	2	16	11	0
Caramel ice cream	89	1 scoop	2	12	4	low

Food	kCalories per portion	Portion size	Protein g	Carbohydrate g	Fat g	Fibre
Caramel shortcake	171	1 slice	1	20	9	low
Caramel toffees	29	1 toffee	trace	6	1	0
Caramel wafers	113	1 standard bar	1	17	5	low
Carbonara pasta sauce	163	¼ jar	2	5	20	0
Carob bar	470	1 standard bar	7	49	27	high
Carpaccio of beef	61	2 thin slices	10	0	2	0
Carrot	35	1 large carrot	1	8	trace	medium
Carrot and orange soup	78	2 ladlefuls	1	12	3	medium
Carrot cake	260	1 slice	3	47	7	medium
Carrot juice	24	1 small glass	trace	6	trace	0
Carrots, honey-glazed	39	3 heaped tablespoons	1	9	trace	medium
Carrots, steamed or boiled	24	3 heaped tablespoons	1	5	trace	medium
Cashew nuts, fresh	143	25 g/1 oz/¼ cup	5	4	12	high
Cashew nuts, roasted	92	1 small handful	3	3	8	high
Cassata	227	1 serving	3	14	23	low
Cassava, baked	310	1 serving	2	80	trace	high
Cassava, boiled	130	1 serving	trace	33	trace	high
Cassoulet	341	1 serving	21	38	13	high
Castle pudding	233	1 individual pudding	3	36	2	medium
Catfish, fried (sautéed), in breadcrumbs	265	1 piece of fillet	21	9	15	low
Catfish, grilled (broiled)	217	1 piece of fillet	27	0	2	0

Food	kCalories per portion	Portion size	Protein g	Carbo-hydrate g	Fat g	Fibre
Catfish, steamed or poached	141	1 piece of fillet	31	0	2	0
Catsup See Ketchup						
Cauliflower	34	4 medium florets	4	3	1	medium
Cauliflower, in white sauce, made with semi-skimmed milk	124	3 heaped tablespoons	6	10	7	medium
Cauliflower, in white sauce, made with skimmed milk	114	3 heaped tablespoons	6	10	6	medium
Cauliflower, steamed or boiled	28	4 medium florets	3	2	1	medium
Cauliflower bhaji	150	1 bhaji	3	3	14	medium
Cauliflower cheese	157	1 serving	9	8	10	medium
Cauliflower soup	133	2 ladlefuls	7	16	5	medium
Caviar, red or black	40	1 tablespoon	4	1	3	0
Celeriac (celery root)	20	¼ small head	1	3	trace	high
Celeriac, steamed or boiled	15	3 heaped tablespoons	1	2	trace	high
Celery	2	1 stick	trace	trace	trace	low
Celery, braised	8	4 tablespoons	trace	1	trace	medium
Celery root See Celeriac						
Celery soup, cream of, canned	86	2 ladlefuls	2	7	6	low
Celery soup, packet	50	2 ladlefuls	2	8	2	low
Celery soup, home-made	82	2 ladlefuls	5	11	2	medium
Cellophane noodles, boiled	251	1 serving	2	57	trace	low
Ceps mushrooms, stewed	6	2 tablespoons	1	trace	trace	low

Food	kCalories per portion	Portion size	Protein g	Carbo-hydrate g	Fat g	Fibre
Cereal bars, chewy, all flavours	**131** (average)	1 bar	1	21	5	medium
Cereal bars, crunchy, all flavours	**146** (average)	1 bar	2	17	7	medium
Cervelat	**77**	1 slice	4	trace	7	0
Champagne	**114**	1 wine glass	trace	2	0	0
Channa dahl	**125**	3 heaped tablespoons	5	10	6	high
Chanterelle mushrooms, stewed	**6**	2 tablespoons	1	trace	trace	low
Chantilly cream	**72**	1 tablespoon	trace	trace	8	0
Chapattis, made with fat	**164**	1 chapatti	4	24	6	medium
Chapattis, made without fat	**101**	1 chapatti	4	22	trace	medium
Charentais melon	**57**	½ melon	2	13	trace	medium
Chargrilled chicken sandwiches	**401**	1 round	25	29	20	medium
Chargrilled chicken breast	**192**	1 breast	38	0	4	0
Charlotte russe	**307**	1 serving	6	50	10	low
Chasseur sauce	**36**	5 tablespoons	1	7	trace	0
Chaumes cheese	**94**	1 small wedge	6	trace	8	0
Cheddar cheese	**103**	1 small wedge	6	trace	9	0
Cheddar cheese, low-fat	**65**	1 small wedge	8	trace	4	0
Cheddars	**21**	1 biscuit (cookie)	trace	2	1	low
Cheerios, dry	**92**	25 g/1 oz/½ cup	2	18	1	medium

Food	kCalories per portion	Portion size	Protein g	Carbo-hydrate g	Fat g	Fibre
Cheerios, with semi-skimmed milk	204	5 heaped tablespoons	7	36	3	medium
Cheerios, with skimmed milk	188	5 heaped tablespoons	7	36	1	medium
Cheese, fresh, soft, full-fat	39	1 tablespoon	1	trace	4	0
Cheese, fresh, soft, low-fat	15	1 tablespoon	1	trace	trace	0
Cheese, fresh, soft, medium-fat	22	1 tablespoon	1	trace	2	0
Cheese, potted	267	1 individual pot	12	1	23	0
See also individual names, e.g. Cheddar						
Cheese and bean enchiladas	547	2 enchiladas	28	82	14	high
Cheese and beef enchiladas	644	2 enchiladas	24	60	36	low
Cheese and coleslaw sandwiches	440	1 round	12	36	28	medium
Cheese and ham sandwiches	432	1 round	19	34	27	medium
Cheese and onion quiche	396	1 slice	14	24	28	medium
Cheese and pickle sandwiches	407	1 round	12	34	26	medium
Cheese and pineapple chunks	25	1 stick	1	1	2	low
Cheese and tomato pizza, deep-pan	300	1 slice	15	30	14	medium
Cheese and tomato pizza, thin-crust	235	1 slice	9	25	12	medium

Food	kCalories per portion	Portion size	Protein g	Carbo-hydrate g	Fat g	Fibre
Cheese and tomato sandwiches	410	1 round	9	11	13	medium
Cheese fondue	492	1 serving	30	8	29	0
Cheese fondue, with French bread	762	1 serving plus 10 cubes of bread	40	62	31	low
Cheese footballs	13	1 football	trace	1	1	low
Cheese melt biscuits (cookies)	21	1 biscuit	trace	3	1	low
Cheese melt biscuits, mini	6	1 biscuit	trace	1	trace	low
Cheese omelette	356	2 eggs	21	trace	30	0
Cheese on toast	223	1 slice	10	21	13	low
Cheese pudding	292	1 serving	17	24	14	low
Cheese sandwiches	398	1 round	12	34	26	medium
Cheese sauce, made with semi-skimmed milk	134	5 tablespoons	6	7	10	low
Cheese sauce, made with skimmed milk	124	5 tablespoons	6	7	8	low
Cheese scone (biscuit)	175	1 scone	5	21	9	low
Cheese scone, with butter	249	1 scone	5	21	17	low
Cheese scone, with low-fat spread	214	1 scone	6	21	13	low
Cheese slice, processed	65	1 slice	4	trace	5	0
Cheese soufflé	280	1 serving	13	10	9	low
Cheese soup, canned	126	2 ladlefuls	4	8	8	low

Food	kCalories per portion	Portion size	Protein g	Carbo-hydrate g	Fat g	Fibre
Cheese soup, home-made	94	2 ladlefuls	6	11	3	low
Cheese spread	41	1 tablespoon	2	1	3	0
Cheese spread, low-fat	27	1 tablespoon	2	1	2	0
Cheese spread, flavoured	35	1 tablespoon	2	1	3	low
Cheese straws	28	1 straw	1	2	trace	low
Cheeseburger	299	1 burger in a bun	16	33	11	medium
Cheesecake, plain, cooked	490	1 slice	4	30	27	low
Cheesecake, plain, set	272	1 slice	5	30	13	low
Cheesecake, with fruit topping	302	1 slice	7	41	13	low
See also *individual flavours*, e.g. Chocolate cheesecake						
Cheeselets	147	1 small bag	3	16	8	medium
Chelsea bun	329	1 bun	7	50	12	medium
Cherries	20	10 cherries	trace	4	trace	low
Cherries, canned in natural juice	51	3 heaped tablespoons	trace	13	trace	low
Cherries, canned in syrup	71	3 heaped tablespoons	trace	18	trace	low
Cherries, glacé (candied)	13	1 cherry	trace	4	trace	low
Cherries, in brandy/kirsch	126	3 heaped tablespoons	trace	18	trace	low
Cherries, maraschino	12	1 cherry	trace	3	trace	low
Cherry bakewells	206	1 individual cake	2	32	8	low
Cherry brandy	64	1 single measure	trace	8	0	0

Food	kCalories per portion	Portion size	Protein g	Carbo-hydrate g	Fat g	Fibre
Cherry cheesecake	**302**	1 slice	7	41	13	low
Cherry compôte	**78**	3 heaped tablespoons	1	20	trace	low
Cherry genoa cake	**334**	1 slice	4	51	12	medium
Cherry pie	**282**	1 slice	3	40	13	medium
Cherry pie filling	**82**	¼ large can	trace	21	trace	low
Cherryade	**18**	1 tumbler	trace	21	trace	0
Cheshire cheese	**94**	1 small wedge	6	trace	8	0
Chestnut purée, sweetened	**45**	1 tablespoon	trace	10	trace	medium
Chestnut purée, unsweetened	**25**	1 tablespoon	trace	5	trace	medium
Chestnut stuffing	**58**	1 serving	1	4	4	medium
Chestnuts	**18**	1 nut	trace	4	trace	high
Chestnuts, peeled and cooked	**65**	5 nuts	1	14	trace	high
Chestnuts, roasted in shells	**21**	1 nut	trace	4	trace	high
Chèvre cheese	**80**	1 small wedge	5	trace	7	0
Chewy cereal bars, all flavours	**131** (average)	1 bar	1	21	5	medium
Chick pea dahl	**125**	3 heaped tablespoons	5	10	6	high
Chick pea goulash	**338**	1 serving	12	36	15	high
Chick peas (garbanzos), canned, drained	**115**	3 heaped tablespoons	7	16	3	high
Chick peas, dried, soaked and boiled	**121**	3 heaped tablespoons	8	18	2	high
Chicken, breast, cooked, sliced	**35**	1 slice	7	0	1	0

Food	kCalories per portion	Portion size	Protein g	Carbohydrate g	Fat g	Fibre
Chicken, breast, grilled (broiled)	213	1 medium breast	40	0	6	0
Chicken, breast, poached or steamed	244	1 medium breast	44	0	7	0
Chicken, breast, smoked	23	1 slice	2	trace	1	0
Chicken, breast portion, fried (sautéed), in breadcrumbs	363	¼ small chicken	27	22	19	low
Chicken, drumstick, barbecued	103	1 drumstick	16	2	4	0
Chicken, drumstick, roast	92	1 drumstick	15	0	3	0
Chicken, fried	494	2 pieces	36	19	29	low
Chicken, jerk	256	1 serving	32	15	8	high
Chicken, leg portion, barbecued	287	¼ small chicken	46	1	10	0
Chicken, leg portion, grilled	274	¼ small chicken	46	0	10	0
Chicken, leg portion, roast	276	¼ small chicken	46	0	10	0
Chicken, lemon	356	1 medium breast	58	3	13	0
Chicken, minced (ground), stewed	183	1 serving	29	0	7	0
Chicken, roast, with skin	216	3 medium slices	23	0	14	0
Chicken, roast, without skin	148	3 medium slices	25	0	5	0
Chicken, steamed	197	¼ small chicken	29	7	4	low
Chicken, sweet and sour	165	1 serving	6	32	2	high

Food	kCalories per portion	Portion size	Protein g	Carbo-hydrate g	Fat g	Fibre
Chicken, tandoori	375	¼ small chicken	47	4	19	trace
Chicken, thai, with noodles	506	1 serving	34	59	15	high
Chicken, wing portion, grilled (broiled)	220	¼ small chicken	36	0	9	0
Chicken, wing portion, roast	222	¼ small chicken	36	0	9	0
Chicken, wings, barbecued, Chinese-style	70	1 wing	9	3	2	0
Chicken à la king	255	1 serving	23	20	9	medium
Chicken and almond soup, canned	180	2 ladlefuls	5	9	14	low
Chicken and sweetcorn (corn) chowder, home-made	183	2 ladlefuls	25	16	3	medium
Chicken and sweetcorn soup, canned	84	2 ladlefuls	3	12	2	low
Chicken and sweetcorn soup, instant	119	1 mug	1	16	6	low
Chicken and ham paste	56	1 tablespoon	4	trace	4	0
Chicken and ham pie, cold	380	1 slice	12	32	22	low
Chicken and mushroom casserole	413	1 serving	39	29	16	low
Chicken and mushroom chowder	192	1 serving	7	17	10	low
Chicken and mushroom pie	246	1 individual pie	16	17	12	low

Food	kCalories per portion	Portion size	Protein g	Carbohydrate g	Fat g	Fibre
Chicken and mushroom soup, canned	76	2 ladlefuls	2	7	4	low
Chicken and mushroom soup, instant	58	1 mug	1	9	2	low
Chicken and rice soup, canned	82	2 ladlefuls	1	15	2	low
Chicken and rice soup, home-made	127	2 ladlefuls	12	13	3	low
Chicken and tarragon soup, home-made	116	2 ladlefuls	3	9	8	low
Chicken and vegetable soup, canned	82	2 ladlefuls	4	12	2	medium
Chicken and vegetable soup, home-made	165	2 ladlefuls	12	19	5	high
Chicken and vegetable stir-fry	270	1 serving	22	39	7	high
Chicken broth	64	2 ladlefuls	2	11	2	low
Chicken burger in a bun, home-made, with relish	366	1 burger in a bun	38	32	10	medium
Chicken burger sandwich	710	1 burger	26	54	43	medium
Chicken byriani	782	1 serving	18	75	38	medium
Chicken cacciatore	265	1 serving	22	36	4	high
Chicken casserole	374	1 serving	38	29	12	high
Chicken chasseur	440	1 serving	27	67	7	medium

Food	kCalories per portion	Portion size	Protein g	Carbo-hydrate g	Fat g	Fibre
Chicken chop suey	**295**	1 serving	23	34	6	medium
Chicken chow mein	**337**	1 serving	22	28	5	high
Chicken cordon bleu	**344**	1 serving	25	15	20	low
Chicken curry, home-made	**615**	1 serving	31	9	51	medium
Chicken curry, home-made, with rice	**863**	1 serving	36	65	53	medium
Chicken curry, retail	**447**	1 serving	36	16	27	medium
Chicken curry, retail, with rice	**691**	1 serving	37	68	26	high
Chicken enchiladas	**566**	2 enchiladas	32	66	9	high
Chicken fajitas	**258**	2 fajitas	16	34	6	low
Chicken fingers	**27**	1 finger	4	2	1	low
Chicken fricassée	**280**	1 serving	28	6	16	medium
Chicken galantine	**268**	1 slice	26	9	14	medium
Chicken goujons	**162**	1 serving	24	12	3	low
Chicken in black bean sauce	**221**	1 serving	29	10	6	medium
Chicken jalfrezi	**490**	1 serving	26	70	12	high
Chicken kiev	**473**	1 medium breast	28	22	31	low
Chicken korma	**460**	1 serving	54	16	21	medium
Chicken liver pâté	**158**	1 serving	6	trace	14	0
Chicken liver pâté, with toast and butter	**468**	1 serving plus 2 slices of toast	13	37	32	medium
Chicken liver risotto	**590**	1 serving	13	89	27	low

Food	kCalories per portion	Portion size	Protein g	Carbo-hydrate g	Fat g	Fibre
Chicken livers, fried (sautéed)	194	1 serving	21	3	11	0
Chicken marsala	284	1 serving	27	2	5	low
Chicken maryland	484	¼ small chicken	36	30	25	low
Chicken mayonnaise sandwiches	458	1 round	12	34	41	medium
Chicken noodle soup, canned	50	2 ladlefuls	3	8	trace	low
Chicken noodle soup, home-made	145	2 ladlefuls	10	17	4	low
Chicken noodle soup, packet	40	2 ladlefuls	2	7	1	low
Chicken nuggets	253	6 nuggets	19	11	15	medium
Chicken omelette	293	2 eggs	21	trace	23	0
Chicken paprika	194	1 serving	31	6	7	low
Chicken paste	35	1 tablespoon	2	trace	3	0
Chicken pie, individual	378	1 individual pie	12	30	22	low
Chicken pie, with puff pastry (paste)	572	1 serving	23	36	37	low
Chicken pot pie	485	1 slice	17	28	39	low
Chicken pot roast with vegetables	510	1 serving	37	65	11	high
Chicken ravioli	148	1 serving	7	26	1	medium
Chicken risotto	336	1 serving	31	83	8	low
Chicken roll, sliced	22	1 slice	3	trace	1	0
Chicken salad	215	1 serving	32	5	7	high

Food	kCalories per portion	Portion size	Protein g	Carbo-hydrate g	Fat g	Fibre
Chicken salad, dressed	318	1 serving	33	5	19	high
Chicken sandwiches	341	1 round	12	5	23	medium
Chicken satay	172	1 stick	26	6	5	low
Chicken soup, cream of, canned	116	2 ladlefuls	3	9	8	0
Chicken soup, home-made	114	2 ladlefuls	12	7	4	0
Chicken soup, instant	100	1 mug	1	11	6	0
Chicken soup, low-fat, canned	44	2 ladlefuls	2	4	2	0
Chicken soup, packet	128	2 ladlefuls	2	21	5	0
Chicken stew with dumplings	537	1 serving	38	77	9	high
Chicken suprême	309	1 breast	43	8	12	low
Chicken tenders	350	8 pieces	22	17	22	low
Chicken teriyaki	317	1 serving	19	52	4	high
Chicken tikka	369	1 serving	43	11	17	medium
Chicken tikka masala	490	1 serving	38	44	18	high
Chicken véronique	254	1 serving	27	11	10	low
Chicken vindaloo	572	1 serving	48	7	40	medium
Chicory (Belgian endive)	18	1 head	2	trace	2	low
Chicory, braised	38	1 head	3	2	2	low
Chilli beans	247	1 serving	15	52	2	high
Chilli con carne	302	1 serving	22	17	17	high

Food	kCalories per portion	Portion size	Protein g	Carbo- hydrate g	Fat g	Fibre
Chilli dog	**204**	1 dog in a bun	7	29	7	low
Chilli salsa	**18**	1 tablespoon	trace	4	trace	low
Chilli sauce	**15**	1 tablespoon	trace	3	trace	low
Chinese egg noodles, cooked	**124**	1 serving	4	26	1	medium
Chinese leaves (stem lettuce)	**11**	1 serving	1	1	0	low
Chinese pork spare ribs	**310**	2 ribs	25	13	17	low
Chipolata sausages, fried (sautéed)	**61**	1 sausage	3	2	5	low
Chipolata sausages, grilled (broiled)	**58**	1 sausage	3	2	5	low
Chips (fries), chip-shop	**394**	1 serving	5	49	20	high
Chips, crinkle-cut, frozen, deep-fried	**478**	1 serving	6	55	27	high
Chips, home-made, deep-fried	**312**	1 serving	6	50	11	high
Chips, microwave	**221**	1 small box	4	32	10	high
Chips, oven, frozen, baked	**267**	1 serving	5	49	7	high
Chips, straight-cut, frozen, deep-fried	**450**	1 serving	6	53	16	high
Chips, thin-cut	**462**	1 serving	5	56	26	high
See also French fries						
Choc ice, any chocolate	**180**	1 ice cream	2	18	11	low
Choco corn flakes, dry	**95**	25 g/1 oz/½ cup	1	21	1	low

Food	kCalories per portion	Portion size	Protein g	Carbo-hydrate g	Fat g	Fibre
Choco corn flakes, with semi-skimmed milk	209	5 heaped tablespoons	6	35	3	low
Choco corn flakes, with skimmed milk	193	5 heaped tablespoons	6	35	1	low
Chocolate, milk	255	1 standard bar	4	28	14	0
Chocolate, plain (semi-sweet)	250	1 standard bar	2	30	13	0
Chocolate, white	109	1 standard (thin) bar	2	11	6	0
Chocolate, with fruit and nut	240	1 standard bar	4	27	12	0
Chocolate, with whole nuts	270	1 standard bar	5	24	17	0
Chocolate and walnut brownies	505	1 brownie	7	40	37	medium
Chocolate biscuits (cookies), full-coated	131	1 biscuit	1	17	7	low
Chocolate biscuits, half-coated	84	1 biscuit	1	11	4	low
Chocolate brazils	49	1 sweet (candy)	1	3	4	high
Chocolate brownies	368	1 brownie	5	63	11	medium
Chocolate buttons	175	1 small packet	3	19	10	0
Chocolate cake, chocolate-coated	268	1 slice	3	41	10	low
Chocolate cake, filled with butter cream	235	1 slice	3	35	10	low
Chocolate caramels	25	1 sweet (candy)	trace	6	trace	low
Chocolate cheesecake	271	1 slice	12	34	11	low

Food	kCalories per portion	Portion size	Protein g	Carbo-hydrate g	Fat g	Fibre
Chocolate chip chewy cereal bar	112	1 bar	1	17	4	low
Chocolate chip cookies	45	1 cookie	trace	8	1	low
Chocolate chip ice cream	91	1 scoop	2	12	4	low
Chocolate chip muffin	397	1 muffin	5	51	22	low
Chocolate corn pops, dry	97	25 g/1 oz/½ cup	1	20	1	low
Chocolate corn pops, with semi-skimmed milk	213	5 heaped tablespoons	6	38	4	low
Chocolate corn pops, with skimmed milk	197	5 heaped tablespoons	6	38	2	low
Chocolate cream biscuits (cookies)	63	1 biscuit	1	9	3	low
Chocolate cream pie	343	1 slice	3	38	22	low
Chocolate crispix, dry	90	25 g/1 oz/½ cup	1	21	1	low
Chocolate crispix, with semi-skimmed milk	201	5 heaped tablespoons	6	40	3	low
Chocolate crispix, with skimmed milk	185	5 heaped tablespoons	6	40	1	low
Chocolate custard, canned	71	¼ large can	2	11	2	low
Chocolate dessert	136	1 individual pot	2	19	5	low
Chocolate dessert, with cream	225	1 individual pot	4	24	12	low
Chocolate digestives (graham crackers)	88	1 biscuit (cookie)	1	11	4	medium
Chocolate éclair toffees	48	1 toffee	trace	7	2	low

Food	kCalories per portion	Portion size	Protein g	Carbo-hydrate g	Fat g	Fibre
Chocolate éclair, filled with cream	277	1 éclair	4	18	21	low
Chocolate éclair, filled with custard	262	1 éclair	6	24	16	low
Chocolate finger biscuits (cookies)	38	1 biscuit	trace	5	2	low
Chocolate fudge	65	1 piece	trace	13	1	low
Chocolate fudge cake	420	1 slice	5	70	14	low
Chocolate fudge fingers	135	1 finger	1	22	5	0
Chocolate fudge icing (frosting)	77	1 tablespoon	trace	9	1	low
Chocolate ginger	30	1 piece	trace	7	trace	low
Chocolate ice cream	89	1 scoop	2	12	4	low
Chocolate layer cake	384	1 slice	5	58	14	low
Chocolate mini roll	119	1 roll	1	16	5	low
Chocolate mint creams	39	1 mint	trace	8	1	0
Chocolate mousse	139	1 individual pot	4	20	5	0
Chocolate mousse, low-calorie	88	1 individual pot	0	0	3	0
Chocolate nut sundae	417	1 sundae	4	52	23	low
Chocolate peanuts	200	1 small packet	5	19	13	medium
Chocolate pot	136	1 individual pot	2	19	5	low
Chocolate profiteroles	373	1 serving	6	33	24	medium
Chocolate pudding	340	1 serving	6	45	16	medium

Food	kCalories per portion	Portion size	Protein g	Carbo-hydrate g	Fat g	Fibre
Chocolate raisins	185	1 small packet	2	32	7	high
Chocolate ripple ice-cream	89	1 scoop	2	12	4	low
Chocolate roulade	206	1 serving	4	20	12	0
Chocolate sauce, for ice cream	192	2 tablespoons	5	29	6	low
Chocolate sauce, made with semi-skimmed milk	112	5 tablespoons	3	14	5	low
Chocolate sauce, made with skimmed milk	102	5 tablespoons	3	14	4	low
Chocolate shreddies, dry	91	25 g/1 oz/½ cup	2	20	trace	medium
Chocolate shreddies, with semi-skimmed milk	224	5 heaped tablespoons	8	42	3	high
Chocolate shreddies, with skimmed milk	208	5 heaped tablespoons	8	42	1	high
Chocolate soufflé	103	1 serving	7	17	1	low
Chocolate soya ice dessert	52	1 scoop	1	5	3	0
Chocolate spread, all types	82 (average)	1 tablespoon	1	9	5	low
Chocolate spread, with peanut butter	89	1 tablespoon	2	5	7	medium
Chocolate wafer bar	115	1 standard bar	1	13	6	0
Chocolates, assorted, filled	46 (average)	1 chocolate	trace	7	2	0
Chorizo sausage	273	1 small sausage	14	1	23	0

Food	kCalories per portion	Portion size	Protein g	Carbo-hydrate g	Fat g	Fibre
Choux buns, filled with cream	**237**	1 bun	4	8	21	low
Choux buns, filled with custard	**293**	1 bun	7	27	17	low
Christmas cake, with marzipan and royal icing (frosting)	**356**	1 slice	4	63	11	medium
Christmas pudding	**291**	1 serving	5	49	10	medium
Ciabatta bread	**125**	1 medium slice	4	26	trace	medium
Cider, dry	**108**	1 small	trace	8	0	0
Cider, medium-sweet	**126**	1 small	trace	13	0	0
Cider, vintage	**303**	1 small	trace	22	0	0
Cider cup	**62**	1 wine glass	trace	17	0	0
Cigarettes russes	**56**	1 biscuit (cookie)	1	6	3	low
Cinnamon danish pastries	**270**	1 pastry	6	52	18	medium
Cinnamon grahams, dry	**102**	25 g/1 oz/½ cup	1	19	2	medium
Cinnamon grahams, with semi-skimmed milk	**182**	3 heaped tablespoons	5	29	5	medium
Cinnamon grahams, with skimmed milk	**166**	3 heaped tablespoons	5	29	3	medium
Clafoutis	**242**	1 serving	7	33	10	medium
Clam bisque, canned	**85**	2 ladlefuls	5	12	2	low
Clam chowder, home-made	**253**	2 ladlefuls	22	17	10	medium

Food	kCalories per portion	Portion size	Protein g	Carbo-hydrate g	Fat g	Fibre
Clams, canned, drained	60	½ medium can	9	2	1	0
Clams, fresh, shelled, cooked	93	1 serving	15	4	1	0
Classic chocolate bar	125	1 standard bar	1	15	7	low
Clear conserve *See Jelly, individual flavours, e.g. Mint jelly, Redcurrant jelly*						
Clementine	28	1 fruit	1	6	trace	medium
Clotted cream fudge	80	1 square	trace	14	3	0
Club chocolate bar, all flavours	125 (average)	1 bar	1	16	7	low
Clusters, dry	97	25 g/1 oz/½ cup	3	17	2	medium
Clusters, with skimmed milk	160	3 heaped tablespoons	7	26	3	medium
Clusters, with semi-skimmed milk	176	3 heaped tablespoons	7	26	5	medium
Cob loaf	70	1 medium slice	3	15	1	low
Cob nuts, shelled	162	25 g/1 oz/¼ cup	3	1	16	medium
Cobbler *See individual flavours, e.g. Fruit cobbler*						
Coca-cola	78	1 tumbler	trace	21	0	0
Coca-cola, diet	1	1 tumbler	0	0	0	0
Cock-a-leekie soup, home-made	138	2 ladlefuls	2	15	8	low
Cockles, fresh, shelled, cooked	48	1 serving	11	trace	trace	0

Food	kCalories per portion	Portion size	Protein g	Carbo-hydrate g	Fat g	Fibre
Cockles, preserved in vinegar	49	1 serving	12	1	trace	0
Cocktail sauce	51	1 tablespoon	trace	2	4	low
Coco pops, dry	95	25 g/1 oz/½ cup	1	21	1	low
Coco pops, with semi-skimmed milk	209	5 heaped tablespoons	5	27	3	low
Coco pops, with skimmed milk	193	5 heaped tablespoons	5	27	1	low
Coco pops cereal and milk bar	90	1 bar	2	14	3	low
Cocoa, made with semi-skimmed milk and sugar	142	1 mug	9	17	5	low
Cocoa, made with skimmed milk and sugar	126	1 mug	9	17	3	low
Coconut	330	¼ nut	3	13	31	high
Coconut, desiccated (shredded)	43	1 tablespoon	1	1	9	high
Coconut cake	175	1 slice	3	20	19	low
Coconut ice sweet (candy) bar	464	1 standard bar	2	83	13	high
Coconut macaroons	117	1 macaroon	1	16	5	medium
Coconut pyramid	230	1 pyramid	1	42	6	high
Coconut rings/thins	35	1 biscuit (cookie)	trace	5	1	low
Cod, baked	168	1 serving	37	0	2	0
Cod, grilled (broiled)	166	1 piece of fillet	36	0	2	0
Cod, fried (sautéed), in batter	497	1 piece of fillet	49	19	26	low

Food	kCalories per portion	Portion size	Protein g	Carbo-hydrate g	Fat g	Fibre
Cod, fried (sautéed), in breadcrumbs	435	1 piece of fillet	53	9	21	low
Cod, salt, soaked and cooked	241	1 piece of fillet	57	0	2	0
Cod, with butter sauce	159	1 steak	18	9	9	low
Cod, with cheese sauce	175	1 steak	20	9	6	low
Cod, with mushroom sauce	168	1 steak	18	9	8	low
Cod, with parsley sauce	170	1 steak	19	11	5	low
Cod and prawn pie	328	1 individual pie	17	24	21	low
Cod mornay	415	1 steak	29	23	23	low
Cod provençal	273	1 serving	39	9	9	medium
Cod roes, in breadcrumbs, fried (sautéed)	202	1 serving	21	3	12	low
Cod roes, on toast	307	1 serving plus 1 slice of toast	20	10	20	low
Coffee, black	5	1 mug	trace	1	trace	0
Coffee, espresso	4	1 small cup	trace	1	trace	0
Coffee, white, made with water and semi-skimmed milk	15	1 mug	1	2	trace	0
Coffee, white, made with water and skimmed milk	12	1 mug	1	2	trace	0
Coffee and walnut cake	344	1 slice	7	34	19	medium
Coffee cake	258	1 slice	5	34	11	low

Food	kCalories per portion	Portion size	Protein g	Carbo-hydrate g	Fat g	Fibre
Coffee cheesecake	272	1 slice	5	30	13	low
Coffee granita	44	1 serving	trace	11	trace	0
Coffee ice cream	89	1 scoop	2	12	4	low
Coffee mousse	139	1 serving	4	20	5	0
Coffee roulade	206	1 slice	4	20	12	0
Coffee streusel cake	263	1 slice	4	29	15	medium
Coffeemate	27	1 teaspoon	trace	3	2	0
Coffeemate, light	21	1 teaspoon	trace	3	1	0
Cointreau	78	1 single measure	trace	7	0	0
Cola	78	1 tumbler	trace	21	0	0
Cola, low-calorie	1	1 tumbler	0	0	0	0
Colcannon	240	1 serving	3	7	18	high
Coleslaw, home-made	92	2 tablespoons	3	13	4	high
Coleslaw, low-calorie	28	2 tablespoons	trace	2	2	medium
Coleslaw, ready-made	40	2 tablespoons	trace	3	3	medium
Coley, fried (sautéed), in batter	490	1 piece of fillet	48	19	25	low
Coley, fried, in breadcrumbs	428	1 piece of fillet	52	9	20	low
Coley, poached or steamed	147	1 piece of fillet	35	0	1	0
Collard greens See Spring greens						
Complan, savoury, made with water	194	1 mug	10	24	7	0

Food	kCalories per portion	Portion size	Protein g	Carbo-hydrate g	Fat g	Fibre
Complan, sweet, made with semi-skimmed milk	**260**	1 mug	14	34	9	low
Complan, sweet, made with skimmed milk	**240**	1 mug	14	34	6	low
Complan, sweet, made with water	**192**	1 mug	9	27	6	low
Conchiglie (pasta shapes), dried, boiled	**198**	1 serving	7	42	1	medium
Conchiglie, fresh, boiled	**235**	1 serving	9	45	2	medium
Condensed milk, skimmed, sweetened	**267**	100 ml/3½ fl oz/ scant ½ cup	10	60	trace	0
Condensed milk, skimmed, unsweetened	**80**	100 ml/3½ fl oz/ scant ½ cup	10	11	trace	0
Condensed milk, whole, sweetened	**333**	100 ml/3½ fl oz/ scant ½ cup	8	55	10	0
Condensed milk, whole, unsweetened	**151**	100 ml/3½ fl oz/ scant ½ cup	8	8	9	0
Conger eel, grilled (broiled)	**375**	1 steak	38	0	24	0
Consommé, canned	**14**	2 ladlefuls	3	1	trace	0
Consommé, jellied	**32**	2 ladlefuls	5	2	trace	0
Cookies See Biscuits						
Cook-in sauces, all flavours	**43** (average)	1 serving	1	8	1	low

Food	kCalories per portion	Portion size	Protein g	Carbo-hydrate g	Fat g	Fibre
Coq au vin	410	1 serving	30	7	29	low
Coquilles st jacques	212	1 serving	10	20	10	medium
Cordial See individual flavours, e.g. Blackcurrant cordial						
Corn chips	229	1 small bag	4	30	11	medium
Corn chowder	143	2 ladlefuls	5	28	2	high
Corn cobs, baby, canned, drained	23	4 cobs	3	2	trace	medium
Corn cobs, baby, steamed or boiled	24	4 cobs	2	3	trace	medium
Corn cobs, baby, stir-fried	69	4 cobs	2	3	5	medium
Corn flakes, dry	92	25 g/1 oz/½ cup	2	20	trace	low
Corn flakes, with semi-skimmed milk	149	5 heaped tablespoons	6	27	2	low
Corn flakes, with skimmed milk	133	5 heaped tablespoons	6	27	trace	low
Corn flakes cereal and chocolate milk bar	118	1 bar	2	18	4	low
Corn fritters	91	1 fritter	2	16	2	medium
Corn kernels, canned, drained See also Sweetcorn	122	3 heaped tablespoons	3	27	1	medium
Corn pops, dry	90	25 g/1 oz/½ cup	1	22	trace	low

Food	kCalories per portion	Portion size	Protein g	Carbo-hydrate g	Fat g	Fibre
Corn pops, with semi-skimmed milk	**209**	5 heaped tablespoons	7	38	3	low
Corn pops, with skimmed milk	**193**	5 heaped tablespoons	7	38	1	low
Corn pops, chocolate, dry	**97**	25 g/1 oz/½ cup	1	20	1	low
Corn pops, chocolate, with semi-skimmed milk	**213**	5 heaped tablespoons	6	38	4	low
Corn pops, chocolate, with skimmed milk	**197**	5 heaped tablespoons	6	38	2	low
Corn puff snacks, all flavours	**259** (average)	1 small bag	3	27	16	low
Corn salad	**3**	1 handful	trace	trace	trace	low
Cornbread	**153**	1 piece	4	22	5	medium
Corned beef	**54**	1 slice	7	0	3	0
Corned beef hash	**387**	1 serving	21	22	24	medium
Cornetto, all flavours	**198** (average)	1 cornet	3	26	10	low
Cornflour pudding	**134**	1 serving	6	26	2	low
Cornichons See Gherkins						
Cornish crab soup, canned	**118**	2 ladlefuls	6	25	trace	low
Cornish hen See Poussin						
Cornish ice cream	**80**	1 scoop	1	6	2	0
Cornish pasties	**515**	1 pasty	12	48	32	medium

Food	kCalories per portion	Portion size	Protein g	Carbo-hydrate g	Fat g	Fibre
Cornish wafers	**47**	1 wafer	1	5	3	low
Cornmeal *See* Polenta						
Cornmeal muffins	**154**	1 muffin	4	23	6	low
Cornmeal pancakes	**97**	1 pancake	3	15	3	low
Corn on the cob, steamed or boiled	**99**	1 cob	4	17	2	medium
Corn on the cob, with butter	**173**	1 cob	4	17	10	medium
Corn on the cob, with low-fat spread	**138**	1 cob	4	17	6	medium
Coronation chicken	**266**	1 serving	40	15	5	low
Cottage cheese	**98**	1 small tub	14	2	4	0
Cottage cheese, flavoured	**95**	1 small tub	13	3	4	0
Cottage cheese, low-fat	**78**	1 small tub	13	3	1	0
Cottage cheese, low-fat, flavoured	**75**	1 small tub	12	3	1	0
Cottage loaf	**74**	1 medium slice	3	15	1	low
Cottage pie	**330**	1 serving	24	25	19	medium
Coulibiac	**380**	1 thick slice	12	30	25	low
Country store, dry	**87**	25 g/1 oz/¼ cup	2	17	1	medium
Country store, with semi-skimmed milk	**197**	3 heaped tablespoons	8	33	4	high
Country store, with skimmed milk	**181**	3 heaped tablespoons	8	33	2	high

Food	kCalories per portion	Portion size	Protein g	Carbo-hydrate g	Fat g	Fibre
Courgettes (zucchini), fried (sautéed)	63	3 heaped tablespoons	3	3	5	medium
Courgettes, steamed or boiled	19	3 heaped tablespoons	2	2	trace	medium
Courgettes, stuffed	134	2 halves	5	12	8	medium
Courgettes provençal	69	3 heaped tablespoons	3	8	3	medium
Couscous	177	3 heaped tablespoons	6	29	4	medium
Couscous salad	159	3 heaped tablespoons	5	23	6	high
Crab, dressed	459	1 medium crab	63	17	16	low
Crab, dressed, canned	21	½ small can	3	0	3	0
Crab, white meat	81	½ small can	18	0	1	0
Crab and mayonnaise sandwiches	447	1 round	15	34	29	medium
Crab bisque, home-made	185	2 ladlefuls	6	26	7	low
Crab cakes	93	1 cake	12	trace	4	0
Crab cocktail	102	1 serving	10	7	3	medium
Crab sandwiches	344	1 round	14	34	18	medium
Crabapple jelly (clear conserve)	55	1 tablespoon	trace	13	trace	0
Crabsticks	12	1 stick	2	1	trace	0
Cracked wheat See Bulgar						
Crackerbread	20	1 piece	trace	4	trace	low

Food	kCalories per portion	Portion size	Protein g	Carbo-hydrate g	Fat g	Fibre
Crackers, wholemeal See also Biscuits and individual names, e.g. Ritz	**29**	1 cracker	1	5	1	medium
Crackers, dried	**48**	1 small handful	trace	12	trace	high
Cranberries, stewed with sugar	**70**	3 heaped tablespoons	trace	18	trace	low
Cranberry jelly (clear conserve)	**38**	1 tablespoon	trace	10	0	low
Cranberry juice drink	**104**	1 tumbler	trace	25	0	0
Cranberry juice drink, light	**48**	1 tumbler	trace	11	0	0
Cranberry sauce	**24**	1 tablespoon	trace	6	0	low
Crayfish, boiled	**148**	½ crayfish	30	0	2	0
Cream, aerosol	**46**	1 tablespoon	trace	trace	5	0
Cream, canned	**36**	1 tablespoon	trace	trace	4	0
Cream, clotted	**88**	1 tablespoon	trace	trace	9	0
Cream, double (heavy)	**67**	1 tablespoon	trace	trace	7	0
Cream, half	**22**	1 tablespoon	trace	1	2	0
Cream, single (light)	**30**	1 tablespoon	trace	1	3	0
Cream, soured (dairy sour)	**31**	1 tablespoon	trace	1	3	0
Cream, sweetened, imitation	**28**	1 tablespoon	trace	1	4	0
Cream, whipping	**56**	1 tablespoon	trace	trace	6	0
Cream cake	**337**	1 individual cake	6	43	17	low
Cream cheese	**66**	1 tablespoon	trace	trace	7	0

Food	kCalories per portion	Portion size	Protein g	Carbo-hydrate g	Fat g	Fibre
Cream crackers	39	1 cracker	10	74	13	low
Cream crowdie	691	1 serving	3	14	52	medium
Cream of wheat *See Semolina*						
Cream soda	58	1 tumbler	trace	14	trace	low
Cream soups, canned, all flavours *See also individual entries, e.g. Cream of tomato soup*	110 (average)	2 ladlefuls	2	9	8	low
Crème brûlée	492	1 serving	1	18	50	0
Crème caramel	136	1 individual pot	4	26	2	0
Crème de cassis	65	1 single measure	trace	7	0	0
Crème de menthe	125	1 single measure	0	14	trace	0
Creme egg, chocolate	163	1 egg	2	28	6	0
Crème fraîche	56	1 tablespoon	trace	trace	6	0
Crème fraîche, low-fat	25	1 tablespoon	trace	1	2	0
Crêpe, plain	122	1 crêpe	2	14	7	low
Crêpes suzette	317	2 pancakes	4	28	12	medium
Crispbread, rye	27	1 cracker	1	6	trace	medium
Crispbread, starch-reduced	15	1 cracker	trace	3	trace	low
Crispbread, wheat	35	1 cracker	1	7	trace	low
Crispie cakes	69	1 cake	1	11	3	low

Food	kCalories per portion	Portion size	Protein g	Carbo-hydrate g	Fat g	Fibre
Crisps (potato chips), all flavours	136 (average)	1 small bag	1	12	9	medium
Crisps, low-fat, all flavours	114 (average)	1 small bag	2	16	5	medium
Crispy chicken sandwich	500	1 portion	23	54	27	medium
Crispy chicken strips	300	3 strips	26	18	16	low
Crispy duck with pancakes	665	1 serving plus 6 pancakes	39	32	42	high
Crispy noodles	374	1 serving	4	50	17	low
Crispy vegetable fingers	45	1 finger	1	5	2	low
Croissant, all-butter	185	1 croissant	4	20	10	low
Croissant, apple	144	1 croissant	4	21	5	medium
Croissant, chocolate	236	1 croissant	4	26	13	low
Croissant, mini	140	1 croissant	3	15	8	low
Croissant, raisin	212	1 croissant	4	27	10	medium
Croque monsieur	438	1 round	20	36	27	medium
Croquette potatoes, fried (sautéed)	214	2 croquettes	4	22	13	medium
Croquette potatoes, frozen, baked	90	2 croquettes	2	14	3	low
Crostini, garlic	31	1 slice	1	5	1	low
Crostini, mushroom	92	1 slice	3	16	2	low
Croûtons	75	1 tablespoon	1	7	5	low

Food	kCalories per portion	Portion size	Protein g	Carbo-hydrate g	Fat g	Fibre
Crown roast of lamb	488	1 serving	30	0	40	0
Crudités	35	1 good handful	1	8	0	medium
Crudités, with aioli	272	1 serving	1	8	23	medium
Crumpet	80	1 crumpet	3	10	0	low
Crumpet, toasted, with butter	117	1 crumpet	3	10	4	low
Crumpet, toasted, with low-fat spread	99	1 crumpet	4	10	2	low
Crunchie chocolate bar	195	1 standard bar	2	30	8	0
Crunchy bran, dry	74	25 g/1 oz/½ cup	3	13	1	high
Crunchy bran, with semi-skimmed milk	175	5 heaped tablespoons	9	27	4	high
Crunchy bran, with skimmed milk	159	5 heaped tablespoons	9	27	2	high
Crunchy cereal bars, all flavours	146 (average)	1 bar	2	17	7	medium
Crunchy mixed grain cereal, with nuts and raisins, dry	97	25 g/1 oz/¼ cup	2	16	3	high
Crunchy mixed grain cereal, with nuts and raisins and semi-skimmed milk	250	3 heaped tablespoons	9	37	7	high
Crunchy mixed grain cereal, with nuts and raisins and skimmed milk	234	3 heaped tablespoons	9	37	5	high
Crunchy nut corn flakes, dry	97	25 g/1 oz/½ cup	2	20	1	low

Food	kCalories per portion	Portion size	Protein g	Carbo-hydrate g	Fat g	Fibre
Crunchy nut corn flakes, with semi-skimmed milk	213	5 heaped tablespoons	7	39	3	low
Crunchy nut corn flakes, with skimmed milk	197	5 heaped tablespoons	7	39	1	low
Cucumber	4	5 slices	0	1	0	low
Cucumber and yoghurt soup	78	2 ladlefuls	5	9	3	low
Cucumber sandwiches	308	1 round	5	35	17	medium
Cullen skink	170	2 ladlefuls	13	16	6	low
Cumberland butter	53	1 tablespoon	0	29	22	0
Cumberland sauce	64	1 tablespoon	trace	14	trace	0
Cumberland sausage, fried (sautéed)	317	1 sausage	14	11	24	low
Cupcakes, iced (frosted)	179	1 cake	1	37	3	low
Curaçao	78	1 single measure	trace	7	0	0
Curd cheese	15	1 tablespoon	2	trace	trace	0
Curd, lemon or orange	42	1 tablespoon	trace	9	1	low
Curly endive (frisée)	6	1 good handful	trace	2	trace	medium
Curly kale, steamed or boiled	24	3 heaped tablespoons	2	1	1	medium
Curly wurly chocolate bar	125	1 standard bar	1	20	5	0
Currant bread	72	1 slice	2	13	2	low
Currant bread, with butter	146	1 slice	2	13	10	low
Currant bread, with low-fat spread	111	1 slice	3	13	6	low

Food	kCalories per portion	Portion size	Protein g	Carbo-hydrate g	Fat g	Fibre
Currant bun	**148**	1 bun	4	26	4	medium
Currant bun, with butter	**222**	1 bun	4	26	12	medium
Currant bun, with low-fat spread	**187**	1 bun	4	26	8	medium
Currant cake	**177**	1 slice	2	29	6	medium
Currants	**40**	1 small handful	trace	10	trace	high
Curried beans	**168**	1 small can	10	31	1	high
Curried chicken and rice salad	**390**	1 serving	42	43	6	high
Curried fruit chutney	**19**	1 tablespoon	trace	4	trace	low
Curry sauce	**58**	5 tablespoons	1	5	4	low
Custard, canned/carton	**71**	5 tablespoons	2	11	2	low
Custard, chocolate	**71**	5 tablespoons	2	11	2	low
Custard, egg, baked	**130**	1 serving	6	12	7	0
Custard, made with powder and semi-skimmed milk	**75**	5 tablespoons	3	13	trace	low
Custard, made with powder and skimmed milk	**59**	5 tablespoons	3	13	2	low
Custard apple	**101**	1 fruit	2	25	1	medium
Custard creams	**57**	1 biscuit (cookie)	1	8	3	low
Custard sauce, made with semi-skimmed milk	**62**	5 tablespoons	2	7	2	0

Food	kCalories per portion	Portion size	Protein g	Carbo-hydrate g	Fat g	Fibre
Custard sauce, made with skimmed milk	**52**	5 tablespoons	2	7	1	0
Custard tart	**373**	1 individual tart	8	44	20	medium
Custard-style yoghurt	**161**	1 individual pot	8	3	13	0
Cuttlefish, grilled (broiled)	**278**	1 serving	56	2	2	0

Food	kCalories per portion	Portion size	Protein g	Carbo-hydrate g	Fat g	Fibre
Dab, fried (sautéed) in breadcrumbs	378	1 fish	28	16	23	low
Dab, grilled (broiled)	175	1 fish	35	0	3	0
Daiquiri	111	1 cocktail	trace	4	0	0
Dairy milk chocolate bar	255	1 standard bar	4	28	14	0
Daktyla bread	65	1 medium slice	2	12	1	medium
Damsons	3	1 fruit	trace	1	trace	medium
Damsons, stewed	27	3 heaped tablespoons	1	6	trace	medium
Damsons, stewed with sugar	107	3 heaped tablespoons	1	19	trace	medium
Damson jam (conserve)	39	1 tablespoon	trace	10	0	0
Damson pie	290	1 slice	3	14	39	medium
Dandelion and burdock	56	1 tumbler	0	13	trace	low
Dandelion and burdock, low-calorie	3	1 tumbler	0	0	0	0
Danish apple cake	252	1 slice	3	32	10	high
Danish blue cheese	87	1 small wedge	5	trace	7	0
Danish brown bread	51	1 medium slice	2	10	trace	medium
Danish elbo cheese	86	1 small wedge	6	trace	7	0
Danish lumpfish roe	40	1 tablespoon	4	1	3	0
Danish pastries, all types	374 (average)	1 pastry	6	51	18	medium
Danish toaster bread	65	1 slice	2	12	1	low

Food	kCalories per portion	Portion size	Protein g	Carbo-hydrate g	Fat g	Fibre
Danish toaster bread, toasted, with butter	**129**	1 slice	2	12	9	low
Danish toaster bread, toasted, with low-fat spread	**94**	1 slice	2	12	5	low
Danish white bread	**50**	1 medium slice	2	10	trace	low
Date squares	**170**	1 square	4	32	4	high
Dates	**30**	1 fruit	trace	8	trace	high
Dates, dried	**40**	1 fruit	trace	10	trace	high
Dates, stuffed	**50**	1 fruit	2	12	4	high
Dauphinoise potatoes	**235**	1 serving	14	12	15	medium
Derby cheese	**100**	1 small wedge	6	trace	8	0
Devilled chicken	**309**	1 serving	48	6	12	0
Devilled kidneys	**158**	1 serving	21	2	7	0
Devil's food cake	**255**	1 slice	3	40	8	low
Devils on horseback	**52**	1 roll	1	3	4	low
Dhal	**162**	3 heaped tablespoons	7	21	6	high
Diet coke	**1**	1 tumbler	0	0	0	0
Diet pepsi	**1**	1 tumbler	trace	trace	trace	0
Digestive biscuits (graham crackers)	**73**	1 biscuit (cookie)	1	10	3	low
Digestive caramels, chocolate	**81**	1 biscuit	1	11	4	medium
Digestive creams	**63**	1 biscuit (cookie)	1	8	3	low
Dijon mustard	**8**	1 teaspoon	trace	trace	trace	low

Food	kCalories per portion	Portion size	Protein g	Carbo-hydrate g	Fat g	Fibre
Dill pickled cucumbers	15	1 pickle	trace	3	trace	low
Dim sum, assorted	49 (average)	1 piece	3	6	2	low
Ditali (pasta shapes), dried, boiled	198	1 serving	7	42	1	medium
Ditali, fresh, boiled	235	1 serving	9	45	2	medium
Dogfish, fried (sautéed), in batter	464	1 piece of fillet	29	13	33	low
Dolcelatte cheese	106	1 small wedge	4	trace	10	0
Dolmas	221	2 rolls	18	19	9	high
Donor kebab, in pitta bread	588	1 kebab plus 1 bread	33	32	38	medium
Dorset blue cheese	87	1 small wedge	5	trace	7	0
Double chocolate chip muffin	397	1 muffin	5	48	20	low
Double decker chocolate bar	235	1 bar	3	32	10	0
Double gloucester cheese	101	1 small wedge	6	trace	8	0
Doughnut, apple	243	1 doughnut	4	29	12	low
Doughnut, chocolate	270	1 doughnut	3	26	18	medium
Doughnut, cream	265	1 doughnut	4	43	15	low
Doughnut, iced (frosted)	286	1 doughnut	4	42	12	low
Doughnut, jam (jelly)	252	1 doughnut	4	37	11	low
Doughnut, mini	59	1 doughnut	1	7	3	low
Doughnut, plain, ring	236	1 doughnut	4	27	12	low

Food	kCalories per portion	Portion size	Protein g	Carbo-hydrate g	Fat g	Fibre
Dover sole, fried (sautéed), in seasoned flour	342	1 medium fish	25	8	13	low
Dover sole, grilled (broiled)	202	1 medium fish	29	0	9	0
Dr pepper soft drink	78	1 tumbler	trace	21	0	0
Dr pepper, diet	1	1 tumbler	0	0	0	0
Drambuie	85	1 single measure	trace	7	0	0
Dream topping, made with semi-skimmed milk	75	3 heaped tablespoons	2	5	6	low
Dream topping, made with skimmed milk	66	3 heaped tablespoons	2	5	4	low
Dream topping, sugar-free, made with semi-skimmed milk	75	3 heaped tablespoons	3	5	5	low
Dream topping, sugar-free, made with skimmed milk	70	3 heaped tablespoons	3	5	3	0
Dressed crab	459	1 medium crab	63	17	16	low
Dressed crab, canned	21	½ small can	3	0	3	0
Dried fruit compôte	127	3 heaped tablespoons	2	33	trace	high
Drifter chocolate bar	292	1 standard bar	3	40	13	low
Drinking (sweetened) chocolate, made with semi-skimmed milk	177	1 mug	9	27	5	low
Drinking chocolate, made with skimmed milk	146	1 mug	9	27	1	low

Food	kCalories per portion	Portion size	Protein g	Carbo-hydrate g	Fat g	Fibre
Drinking chocolate, instant, made with water	119	1 mug	3	18	4	low
Drinking yoghurt	124	1 tumbler	6	26	trace	0
Drop scone (small pancake)	44	1 pancake	1	6	2	low
Dry-cured Belgian ham	21	1 slice	4	0	1	0
Dry-roasted peanuts	88	1 small handful	4	1	7	high
Dublin bay prawns (saltwater crayfish), cooked	10	1 prawn	2		trace	0
Dubonnet, red	75	1 double measure	trace	8	0	0
Duchesse potatoes	165	2 pieces	5	17	5	medium
Duck, breast, grilled (broiled), without skin	378	1 breast	50	0	19	0
Duck, breast, grilled, with skin	678	1 breast	37	0	58	0
Duck, crispy peking	665	1 serving plus 6 pancakes	39	32	42	high
Duck, roast, with skin	763	¼ duck	44	0	65	0
Duck à l'orange	856	¼ duck	49	8	69	medium
Duck eggs, boiled	106	1 egg	9	trace	8	0
Duck liver pâté	158	1 serving	6	trace	14	0
Duck soup, home-made	114	2 ladlefuls	12	7	4	0
Duck with cherries	836	¼ duck	44	4	65	low
Dumplings	73	1 dumpling	1	9	1	low

Food	kCalories per portion	Portion size	Protein g	Carbo-hydrate g	Fat g	Fibre
Dundee cake	397	1 slice	6	58	17	medium
Dunlop cheese	103	1 small wedge	6	trace	9	0
Dutch apple tart	237	1 slice	3	34	10	medium

Food	kCalories per portion	Portion size	Protein g	Carbo-hydrate g	Fat g	Fibre
Easter biscuits (cookies)	58	1 biscuit	1	16	4	low
Eccles cake	214	1 cake	2	26	12	medium
Echo chocolate bar	132	1 standard bar	2	15	7	low
Eclair, chocolate	277	1 éclair	4	18	21	low
Edam (dutch) cheese	83	1 small wedge	6	trace	6	0
Eel pie mash, with pea gravy	434	1 serving	17	35	25	medium
Eels, jellied	70	1 small serving	6	trace	6	0
Eels, silver, stewed	320	1 serving	25	0	13	0
Eels, smoked	167	1 serving	10	0	13	0
Egg, baked, with cream	151	1 egg	7	trace	13	0
Egg, boiled	84	1 egg	7	trace	6	0
Egg, coddled	84	1 egg	7	trace	6	0
Egg, curried	226	2 eggs	15	5	16	low
Egg, fried (sautéed)	102	1 egg	8	trace	8	0
Egg, pickled	84	1 egg	7	trace	6	0
Egg, poached	84	1 egg	7	trace	6	0
Egg, scotch	301	1 egg	14	16	20	low
Egg, scrambled	308	2 eggs	13	1	28	0
Egg, stuffed	187	2 halves	7	trace	17	0
Egg and cress sandwiches	392	1 round	13	68	23	medium
Egg custard tart	373	1 individual tart	8	44	20	medium
Egg custard, baked	130	1 serving	6	12	7	0

Food	kCalories per portion	Portion size	Protein g	Carbo-hydrate g	Fat g	Fibre
Egg custard, packet, made up with semi-skimmed milk	168	1 serving	5	23	6	0
Egg custard, packet, made up with skimmed milk	149	1 serving	5	23	4	0
Egg fried rice	374	1 serving	7	46	19	low
Egg mayonnaise	290	1 egg	7	trace	29	0
Egg mayonnaise sandwiches	491	1 round	13	34	34	medium
Egg mcmuffin	290	1 portion	17	27	12	medium
Egg nog	68	1 single measure	1	7	2	0
Egg noodles, chinese	124	1 serving	4	26	1	medium
Egg salad	200	2 eggs	16	5	12	high
Egg salad, dressed	297	2 eggs	16	5	29	high
Egg sauce	117	5 tablespoons	5	8	7	low
Eggplant See Aubergine						
Eggs benedict	402	1 egg	22	43	17	medium
Eggs florentine	239	1 egg	16	7	16	medium
Eggy bread	213	1 slice	6	17	18	low
Elderflower pressé	50	1 wine glass	trace	12	trace	0
Elmlea cream blend, double (heavy)	61	1 tablespoon	trace	trace	6	low
Elmlea, single (light)	48	1 tablespoon	trace	trace	5	low
Elmlea, whipping	43	1 tablespoon	trace	trace	4	low
Elmlea light, double (heavy)	37	1 tablespoon	trace	1	4	low

Food	kCalories per portion	Portion size	Protein g	Carbo-hydrate g	Fat g	Fibre
Elmlea light, single (light)	17	1 tablespoon	trace	trace	3	low
Elmlea light, whipping	28	1 tablespoon	trace	trace	2	low
Emmental (swiss) cheese	105	1 small wedge	7	1	8	0
Enchiladas See individual fillings, e.g. Cheese enchiladas						
English muffin	127	1 muffin	5	27	1	medium
English muffin, toasted, with butter	200	1 muffin	5	27	9	medium
English muffin, toasted, with low-fat spread	166	1 muffin	6	27	5	medium
English mustard	7	1 teaspoon	trace	trace	trace	low
Escargots à la bourguignonne	311	6 snails	12	trace	25	low
Escarole	6	1 good handful	trace	2	trace	medium
Esrom cheese	84	1 small wedge	5	trace	7	0
Evaporated milk See Condensed milk, unsweetened						
Everton mints	21	1 mint	trace	4	trace	0
Everton toffee	20	1 toffee	trace	1	0	0
Eve's pudding	222	1 serving	3	40	6	medium
Exotic fruit drink	90	1 tumbler	trace	22	trace	0

Food	kCalories per portion	Portion size	Protein g	Carbohydrate g	Fat g	Fibre
Fab ice lolly	99	1 lolly	1	17	3	0
Faggots	402	2 faggots	16	23	27	low
Fairy cakes	105	1 individual cake	2	22	2	low
Fajitas *See individual fillings, e.g. Beef fajitas*						
Falafels	140	2 falafels	5	11	9	high
Fanta orange	85	1 tumbler	0	22	0	0
Fanta orange, diet	6	1 tumbler	0	0	0	0
Farfalle (pasta shapes), dried, boiled	198	1 serving	7	42	1	medium
Farfalle, fresh, boiled	235	1 serving	9	45	2	medium
Farmhouse loaf	74	1 medium slice	3	15	1	low
Farmhouse vegetable soup, canned	90	2 ladlefuls	4	16	1	medium
Farmhouse vegetable soup, packet	119	2 ladlefuls	4	25	1	high
Feast ice lolly	313	1 lolly	3	23	13	low
Fennel	27	1 head	2	4	3	medium
Fennel, au gratin	145	1 serving	7	8	10	medium
Fennel, steamed or boiled	11	½ head	1	1	trace	medium
Feta cheese	62	1 small chunk	4	trace	5	0
Feta cheese, with olives	19	1 piece of each	1	trace	2	low

Food	kCalories per portion	Portion size	Protein g	Carbo-hydrate g	Fat g	Fibre
Fettuccine (pasta ribbons), dried, boiled	239	1 serving	8	51	2	medium
Fettuccine, fresh, boiled	301	1 serving	11	57	2	medium
Fibre 1, dry	66	25 g/1 oz/½ cup	3	13	1	high
Fibre 1, with semi-skimmed milk	166	5 heaped tablespoons	9	26	3	high
Fibre 1, with skimmed milk	150	5 heaped tablespoons	9	26	1	high
Fig roll biscuit (cookie)	61	1 roll	1	11	2	medium
Figgy duff	581	1 serving	9	80	28	high
Figs	24	1 fig	1	5	trace	high
Figs, canned in syrup	88	3 heaped tablespoons	trace	25	trace	high
Figs, dried, ready-to-eat	45	1 fig	1	11	trace	high
Figs, dried, stewed	103	3 heaped tablespoons	3	29	1	high
Figs, dried, stewed with sugar	143	3 heaped tablespoons	3	34	1	high
Figs, with parma ham	87	1 fig plus 2 slices of ham	9	11	2	high
Filberts *See* Hazelnuts						
Filet-o-fish	389	1 portion	17	41	18	medium
Fillet steak *See* Steak, fillet						
Fingers, milk chocolate	38	1 biscuit (cookie)	trace	6	1	low
Finger rolls	107	1 roll	4	21	2	low
Finnan haddie	148	1 fish	34	0	1	0

Food	kCalories per portion	Portion size	Protein g	Carbo-hydrate g	Fat g	Fibre
Fish and chips, deep-fried, chip-shop-style	**891**	1 serving	54	68	46	high
Fish cakes, salmon, fried (sautéed)	**213**	1 cake	8	15	11	low
Fish cakes, salmon, grilled (broiled)	**192**	1 cake	10	17	7	low
Fish cakes, white fish, fried	**188**	1 cake	9	15	10	low
Fish cakes, white fish, grilled	**169**	1 cake	11	17	6	low
Fish chowder	**285**	2 ladlefuls	44	60	10	medium
Fish fingers, fried (sautéed)	**47**	1 finger	3	3	3	low
Fish fingers, grilled (broiled)	**43**	1 finger	3	4	2	low
Fish goujons	**304**	6 goujons	37	6	14	low
Fish kebabs	**95**	1 kebab	21	0	1	0
Fish mornay	**239**	1 serving	11	13	21	low
Fish mousse	**180**	1 serving	10	6	15	low
Fish paste	**25**	1 tablespoon	2	trace	1	low
Fish pie, topped with pastry (paste)	**384**	1 serving	14	27	25	low
Fish pie, topped with potato	**315**	1 serving	24	37	9	medium
Fish soup	**159**	2 ladlefuls	16	21	2	medium
Fish stew	**330**	1 serving	30	43	5	medium
Fish sticks	**76**	1 stick	4	7	3	0

Food	kCalories per portion	Portion size	Protein g	Carbo-hydrate g	Fat g	Fibre
Flageolet beans, canned, drained	**98**	3 heaped tablespoons	7	21	1	high
Flageolet beans, dried, soaked and cooked	**104**	3 heaped tablespoons	8	23	1	high
Flake chocolate bar	**180**	1 standard bar	3	19	10	0
Flan, fruit, any flavour	**222**	1 slice	3	40	6	low
Flapjack	**417**	1 piece	6	48	23	high
Florida cocktail	**56**	1 serving	trace	10	trace	low
Flounder, fried (sautéed)	**378**	1 small fish	28	16	23	low
Flounder, grilled (broiled)	**175**	1 small fish	35	0	2	0
Focaccia bread	**139**	1 medium slice	3	30	1	medium
Fois gras	**158**	1 serving	6	trace	14	0
Fondant creams	**25**	1 sweet (candy)	trace	7	0	0
Fondant icing (frosting)	**100**	25 g/1 oz	0	25	0	0
Fondue, cheese	**492**	1 serving	30	8	29	0
Fondue, cheese, with French bread	**762**	1 serving plus 10 cubes of bread	40	62	31	medium
Fontina cheese	**110**	1 small wedge	7	trace	9	0
Forcemeat balls	**115**	2 balls	3	10	7	low
Four cheese pizza	**334**	1 slice	13	36	17	medium
Four cheese pasta sauce	**500**	¼ jar	17	76	13	medium
Four seasons pizza	**342**	1 slice	12	32	16	medium
Framboise liqueur	**65**	1 single measure	trace	7	0	0

Food	kCalories per portion	Portion size	Protein g	Carbo-hydrate g	Fat g	Fibre
Frankfurter	186	1 frankfurter	9	2	15	low
Frankfurter, canned	82	1 frankfurter	3	1	7	low
French (green) beans, canned, drained	22	3 heaped tablespoons	1	4	trace	medium
French beans, steamed or boiled	25	3 heaped tablespoons	2	5	trace	high
French dressing	97	1 tablespoon	trace	0	17	0
French dressing, low-calorie	5	1 tablespoon	trace	1	trace	0
French fancies, fondant-iced (frosted)	150	1 cake	1	25	5	low
French fries, thin, from burger outlets See *also* Chips	206	1 serving	3	28	9	medium
French mustard	7	1 teaspoon	trace	1	trace	low
French onion soup, canned	48	2 ladlefuls	2	11	trace	low
French onion soup, home-made	94	2 ladlefuls	2	8	6	low
French onion soup, packet	104	2 ladlefuls	2	20	1	low
French onion soup, with cheese croûtes	226	2 ladlefuls plus 1 croûte	9	21	8	low
French stick	135	1 thick slice	5	27	1	low
French toast	213	1 slice	6	17	18	low
Fried (sautéed) bread	181	1 slice	3	17	11	low

Food	kCalories per portion	Portion size	Protein g	Carbo-hydrate g	Fat g	Fibre
Fried (sautéed) egg sandwiches	406	1 round	13	34	25	medium
Fried rice See Rice, Egg fried rice *and* Special fried rice						
Fries See Chips						
Frisée See Curly endive						
Frito misto	338	1 serving	24	43	11	low
Frittata	328	2 eggs	16	17	22	medium
Frogs' legs, fried (sautéed)	178	2 legs	22	0	10	low
Fromage blanc	12	1 tablespoon	1	trace	trace	0
Fromage frais	113	1 individual pot	7	6	7	0
Fromage frais, flavoured	131	1 individual pot	7	14	6	low
Fromage frais, low-fat	58	1 individual pot	8	7	trace	low
Fromage frais, low-fat, flavoured	58	1 individual pot	8	7	trace	low
Frosted shreddies, dry	91	25 g/1 oz/½ cup	2	20	trace	high
Frosted shreddies, with semi-skimmed milk	224	5 heaped tablespoons	7	43	3	high
Frosted shreddies, with skimmed milk	208	5 heaped tablespoons	7	43	1	high
Frosted wheats, dry	80	25 g/1 oz/½ cup	2	17	trace	high
Frosted wheats, with semi-skimmed milk	185	5 heaped tablespoons	8	34	3	high

Food	kCalories per portion	Portion size	Protein g	Carbo-hydrate g	Fat g	Fibre
Frosted wheats, with skimmed milk	169	5 heaped tablespoons	8	34	1	high
Frosties, dry	95	25 g/1 oz/½ cup	1	22	trace	low
Frosties, with semi-skimmed milk	209	5 heaped tablespoons	6	41	2	low
Frosties, with skimmed milk	193	5 heaped tablespoons	6	41	trace	low
Frosties cereal and milk bar	121	1 bar	3	18	4	low
Frosting *See* Icing						
Fruit cake, light	354	1 slice	5	58	13	medium
Fruit cake, rich *See also* Christmas cake	341	1 slice	4	60	11	medium
Fruit chewy sweets (candies)	185	1 tube	trace	38	4	0
Fruit cobbler	255	1 serving	4	46	7	medium
Fruit cocktail, canned in natural juice	57	3 heaped tablespoons	trace	15	trace	low
Fruit cocktail, canned in syrup	77	3 heaped tablespoons	trace	20	trace	low
Fruit corner yoghurt dessert	219	1 individual carton	6	26	7	low
Fruit flan, made with pastry (paste)	153	1 slice	2	24	6	low
Fruit flan, made with sponge	222	1 slice	3	40	1	low
Fruit gums	134	1 tube	2	32	0	0
Fruit 'n' fibre, dry	87	25 g/1 oz/½ cup	2	17	1	high

Food	kCalories per portion	Portion size	Protein g	Carbo-hydrate g	Fat g	Fibre
Fruit 'n' fibre, with semi-skimmed milk	197	5 heaped tablespoons	8	34	4	high
Fruit 'n' fibre, with skimmed milk	181	5 heaped tablespoons	8	34	2	high
Fruit pastilles	147	1 tube	2	35	0	0
Fruit pie	241	1 individual pie	2	39	8	medium
Fruit punch	59	1 wine glass	0	15	0	low
Fruit salad, canned in natural juice	29	3 heaped tablespoons	trace	7	trace	low
Fruit salad, canned in syrup	57	3 heaped tablespoons	trace	15	trace	low
Fruit salad, dried	145	3 heaped tablespoons	3	40	trace	high
Fruit salad, dried, stewed	83	3 heaped tablespoons	1	26	trace	high
Fruit salad, dried, stewed with sugar	94	3 heaped tablespoons	1	29	trace	high
Fruit salad, fresh, in pure juice	27	3 heaped tablespoons	1	7	trace	medium
Fruit salad, fresh, in syrup	55	3 heaped tablespoons	1	14	trace	medium
Fruit salad, tropical	47	3 heaped tablespoons	1	9	0	medium
Fruit scone (biscuit)	158	1 scone	4	26	5	medium
Fruit scone, with butter	232	1 scone	4	26	13	medium
Fruit scone, with low-fat spread	197	1 scone	5	26	9	medium
Fruit shortcake	52	1 biscuit (cookie)	1	7	2	low

Food	kCalories per portion	Portion size	Protein g	Carbo-hydrate g	Fat g	Fibre
Fruit squash *See individual flavours, e.g. Orange squash*						
Fruitful shredded wheat, dry	88	25 g/1 oz/½ cup	2	17	1	high
Fruitful shredded wheat, with semi-skimmed milk	202	3 heaped tablespoons	8	34	4	high
Fruitful shredded wheat, with skimmed milk	186	3 heaped tablespoons	8	34	2	high
Fruitibix, dry	88	25 g/1 oz/½ cup	2	18	1	high
Fruitibix, with semi-skimmed milk	200	3 heaped tablespoons	8	34	3	high
Fruitibix, with skimmed milk	184	3 heaped tablespoons	8	34	1	high
Fudge *See also individual flavours, e.g. Chocolate fudge*	77	1 square	trace	14	2	0
Fudge brownie	394	1 brownie	5	62	20	low
Ful medames beans, dried, soaked and cooked	116	3 heaped tablespoons	9	20	1	high
Fusilli (pasta spirals), dried, boiled	239	1 serving	8	51	2	medium
Fusilli, fresh, boiled	301	1 serving	11	57	2	medium

Food	kCalories per portion	Portion size	Protein g	Carbohydrate g	Fat g	Fibre
Gaelic coffee	**218**	1 wine glass	1	7	14	0
Gala pie	**564**	1 slice	15	37	68	medium
Galaxy chocolate bar, all flavours	**250** (average)	1 standard bar	4	27	14	0
Galaxy cake bar	**178**	1 cake bar	2	20	10	low
Galaxy cake bar, caramel	**148**	1 cake bar	2	20	7	low
Galaxy double nut and raisin bar	**246**	1 standard bar	4	26	14	0
Galaxy ice cream	**302**	1 ice cream bar	4	28	19	0
Galaxy muffin	**356**	1 muffin	5	42	18	low
Game chips	**273**	10 chips	3	25	19	medium
Game pie	**606**	1 serving	21	49	35	medium
Game soup, canned	**88**	2 ladlefuls	5	10	4	low
Gammon, honey-roast	**174**	2 thick slices	25	4	6	0
Gammon, lean, boiled	**167**	2 thick slices	29	0	5	0
Gammon, rasher (slice), fried (sautéed)	**171**	1 rasher	22	0	9	0
Gammon, rasher, grilled (broiled)	**141**	1 rasher	22	0	8	0
Gammon, steak, grilled	**301**	1 medium steak	54	0	9	0
Gammon with pineapple	**324**	1 medium steak plus 1 pineapple slice	54	6	9	0

Food	kCalories per portion	Portion size	Protein g	Carbo-hydrate g	Fat g	Fibre
Gammon and egg	403	1 medium steak plus 1 egg	62	trace	17	0
Garbanzos See Chick peas						
Garibaldi biscuits (cookies)	41	1 biscuit	trace	7	1	low
Garlic	5	1 clove	trace	1	trace	low
Garlic and herb soft cheese	77	1 good spoonful	2	1	7	low
Garlic bread	73	1 small slice	1	7	4	low
Garlic butter	112	1 tablespoon	trace	trace	12	low
Garlic chicken	316	1 breast	40	3	16	low
Garlic mayonnaise	237	2 tablespoons	trace	trace	23	0
Garlic sausage	12	1 slice	1	trace	1	low
Gazpacho	136	2 ladlefuls	3	trace	7	medium
Genoa cake	383	1 slice	5	56	16	medium
German smoked cheese	60	1 small wedge	4	trace	3	0
Ghee	224	25 g/1 oz/2 tbsp	trace	trace	25	0
Gherkins (cornichons)	4	1 gherkin	trace	1	trace	low
Gin	55	1 single measure	trace	trace	0	0
Gin and dry martini	114	1 cocktail	trace	3	trace	0
Gin and lime	111	1 single measure	trace	15	0	0
Gin and orange	108	1 single measure	trace	7	0	0
Gin and sweet martini	75	1 cocktail	trace	8	0	0

Food	kCalories per portion	Portion size	Protein g	Carbo-hydrate g	Fat g	Fibre
Gin and tonic	76	1 single measure plus 1 mixer	trace	5	0	0
Gin and tonic, low-calorie	56	1 single measure plus 1 mixer	trace	trace	trace	0
Ginger, chocolate	30	1 piece	trace	7	trace	low
Ginger, crystallised	30	1 piece	trace	4	0	low
Ginger, stem, in syrup	30	1 piece	trace	2	trace	low
Ginger ale, american	44	1 tumbler	0	10	0	0
Ginger ale, dry	32	1 tumbler	0	8	0	0
Ginger ale, low-calorie	1	1 tumbler	trace	trace	trace	0
Ginger beer	98	1 tumbler	0	24	0	0
Ginger cake	388	1 slice	3	60	15	medium
Ginger cake bar	128	1 cake bar	1	22	4	low
Ginger ice cream	89	1 scoop	2	11	4	low
Ginger nuts	56	1 biscuit (cookie)	1	9	2	low
Ginger nuts, milk or plain (semi-sweet) chocolate	70	1 biscuit	1	10	3	low
Ginger snaps	37	1 biscuit (cookie)	trace	6	1	low
Ginger wine	200	1 double measure	trace	16	0	0
Gingerbread	180	1 slice	2	28	7	low
Gingerbread men	249	1 man	4	34	11	low
Gipsy creams	64	1 biscuit (cookie)	1	8	3	low
Gjetost cheese	132	1 small wedge	3	12	8	0

Food	kCalories per portion	Portion size	Protein g	Carbo-hydrate g	Fat g	Fibre
Glacé (candied) cherries	**13**	1 cherry	trace	4	trace	low
Glacé (candied) fruits	**13**	1 piece	trace	4	trace	low
Glacé icing (frosting)	**56**	1 tablespoon	0	14	0	0
Globe artichoke, whole, steamed or boiled See also Artichokes	**70**	1 medium artichoke	0	3	0	medium
Globe artichoke heart, canned, drained	**8**	1 heart	1	1	trace	medium
Glucose, powdered or liquid	**48**	1 tablespoon	trace	13	0	0
Gnocchi	**213**	1 serving	3	13	12	low
Gnocchi, with butter and Parmesan	**385**	1 serving	9	13	29	low
Goats' cheese, hard	**128**	1 small wedge	9	1	10	0
Goats' cheese, soft	**76**	1 tablespoon	5	trace	6	0
Goats' milk	**180**	300 ml/½ pt/1¼ cups	9	12	10	0
Golden cutlets (smoked, whiting), poached	**166**	1 medium fillet	21	0	1	0
Golden grahams, dry	**93**	25 g/1 oz/½ cup	1	20	1	low
Golden grahams, with semi-skimmed milk	**172**	5 heaped tablespoons	6	30	3	low
Golden grahams, with skimmed milk	**156**	5 heaped tablespoons	6	30	1	low
Golden nuggets, dry	**95**	25 g/1 oz/½ cup	1	22	trace	low

Food	kCalories per portion	Portion size	Protein g	Carbo-hydrate g	Fat g	Fibre
Golden nuggets, with semi-skimmed milk	**174**	5 heaped tablespoons	6	32	2	low
Golden nuggets, with skimmed milk	**158**	5 heaped tablespoons	6	32	trace	low
Golden raisins *See Sultanas*						
Golden (light corn) syrup	**45**	1 tablespoon	trace	12	0	0
Golden syrup cake bar	**385**	1 cake bar	4	60	14	medium
Golden syrup cake bar, mini	**126**	1 cake bar	1	22	4	low
Goose, roast, without skin	**319**	3 medium slices	29	0	22	0
Gooseberries	**19**	3 heaped tablespoons	1	3	trace	medium
Gooseberries, canned in syrup	**73**	3 heaped tablespoons	trace	18	trace	medium
Gooseberries, stewed	**16**	3 heaped tablespoons	1	2	trace	medium
Gooseberries, stewed with sugar	**54**	3 heaped tablespoons	1	13	trace	medium
Gooseberry fool	**183**	1 serving	3	20	9	medium
Gooseberry pie	**314**	1 slice	4	40	16	medium
Gooseberry sauce	**42**	1 tablespoon	trace	trace	4	medium
Gorgonzola cheese	**106**	1 small wedge	4	trace	10	0
Gouda cheese	**94**	1 small wedge	6	trace	8	0
Gougère, cheese	**239**	1 serving	16	8	24	low
Goulash, hungarian	**406**	1 serving	28	16	22	medium
Graham crackers *See Digestive biscuits*						

Food	kCalories per portion	Portion size	Protein g	Carbohydrate g	Fat g	Fibre
Grainy mustard	7	1 teaspoon	2	1	trace	low
Granary bread	94	1 medium slice	4	18	1	medium
Grand marnier	78	1 single measure	trace	7	0	0
Granda padano cheese	113	1 small wedge	10	trace	8	0
Granola, dry	89	25 g/1 oz/¼ cup	3	17	1	high
Granola, with semi-skimmed milk	236	3 heaped tablespoons	10	40	5	high
Granola, with skimmed milk	226	3 heaped tablespoons	10	40	3	high
Grape juice	92	1 tumbler	1	23	trace	0
Grape juice, red	92	1 tumbler	1	23	trace	0
Grape juice, red, sparkling	61	1 wine glass	trace	16	0	0
Grape juice, white	92	1 tumbler	1	23	trace	0
Grape juice, white, sparkling	61	1 wine glass	trace	16	0	0
Grapefruit	48	1 fruit	2	12	trace	medium
Grapefruit, canned in natural juice	30	3 heaped tablespoons	1	7	trace	low
Grapefruit, canned in syrup	60	3 heaped tablespoons	trace	15	trace	low
Grapefruit, with port	47	½ grapefruit	1	8	trace	medium
Grapefruit, with sugar	64	½ grapefruit	1	16	trace	medium
Grapefruit, with sugar, grilled (broiled)	64	½ grapefruit	1	16	trace	medium
Grapefruit cocktail	72	1 serving	trace	18	trace	low
Grapefruit drink, sparkling	88	1 tumbler	0	24	0	0

Food	kCalories per portion	Portion size	Protein g	Carbo-hydrate g	Fat g	Fibre
Grapefruit juice	66	1 tumbler	1	17	trace	low
Grapefruit juice drink	72	1 tumbler	trace	18	trace	low
Grapenuts, dry	86	25 g/1 oz/½ cup	2	20	trace	medium
Grapenuts, with semi-skimmed milk	195	3 heaped tablespoons	8	26	2	medium
Grapenuts, with skimmed milk	183	3 heaped tablespoons	8	26	trace	medium
Grapes, black	60	1 small bunch	trace	15	trace	low
Grapes, green	60	1 small bunch	trace	15	trace	low
Grappa	79	1 single measure	trace	6	0	0
Gravlax	336	1 serving	34	4	21	0
Gravy, made with giblets or meat juices	56	4 tablespoons	4	2	4	low
Gravy, made with granules	25	4 tablespoons	trace	2	2	low
Gravy, thin	2	4 tablespoons	trace	trace	trace	0
Greek pastries	322	1 piece	5	40	17	medium
Greek slow-roasted lamb See Kleftiko						
Greek pork stew See Afelia						
Greek village salad	108	1 serving	6	5	8	high
Greek-style yoghurt, cows'	161	1 individual pot	8	3	13	0
Greek-style yoghurt, sheep's	149	1 individual pot	6	8	10	0
Greek-style yoghurt, with honey	158	1 serving	6	15	9	0

Food	kCalories per portion	Portion size	Protein g	Carbo-hydrate g	Fat g	Fibre
Green beans See French (green) beans						
Green chartreuse	78	1 single measure	trace	7	0	0
Green salad	14	1 serving	1	2	trace	medium
Green salad, dressed	111	1 serving	1	2	17	medium
Greengage	13	1 fruit	trace	2	trace	medium
Greengage pie	290	1 slice	3	39	14	medium
Greengages, canned in natural juice	51	3 heaped tablespoons	trace	11	trace	medium
Greengages, canned in syrup	69	3 heaped tablespoons	trace	16	trace	medium
Greengages, stewed	37	3 heaped tablespoons	1	6	trace	medium
Greengages, stewed with sugar	117	3 heaped tablespoons	1	19	trace	medium
Grenadine syrup, undiluted	35	1 tablespoon	trace	9	0	0
Griddle scones (biscuits)	44	1 scone	1	6	2	low
Grillsteak, minced (ground) beef, grilled (broiled)	185	1 steak	11	8	12	low
Grillsteak, minced lamb, grilled (broiled)	175	1 steak	14	1	13	0
Ground beef See Beef, minced						
Ground rice pudding, made with semi-skimmed milk	205	1 serving	8	40	11	low

Ground rice pudding

Food	kCalories per portion	Portion size	Protein g	Carbo-hydrate g	Fat g	Fibre
Ground rice pudding, made with skimmed milk	**186**	1 serving	8	40	trace	low
Grouper, grilled (broiled)	**238**	1 piece of fillet	50	6	3	0
Grouse, roast	**456**	1 small bird	82	0	14	0
Gruyère (swiss) cheese	**117**	1 small wedge	8	trace	9	0
Guacamole	**408**	1 serving	1	1	45	medium
Guard of honour, lamb	**340**	1 serving	25	10	22	low
Guava	**26**	1 medium fruit	1	5	trace	high
Guava, canned in natural juice	**48**	3 heaped tablespoons	trace	11	0	high
Guava, canned in syrup	**60**	3 heaped tablespoons	trace	16	0	high
Guinea fowl, roast	**480**	¼ bird	74	0	14	0
Guinness	**117**	1 small	1	6	trace	0

Food	kCalories per portion	Portion size	Protein g	Carbo-hydrate g	Fat g	Fibre
Haddock, fried (sautéed), in batter	**490**	1 piece of fillet	46	19	26	low
Haddock, fried, in breadcrumbs	**435**	1 piece of fillet	53	9	26	low
Haddock, poached or steamed	**171**	1 piece of fillet	40	0	1	0
Haddock, smoked, poached	**176**	1 piece of fillet	41	0	1	0
Haggis	**310**	1 serving	11	19	22	low
Hake, fried (sautéed), in batter	**497**	1 piece of fillet	49	19	26	low
Hake, poached or steamed	**164**	1 piece of fillet	42	0	7	0
Halibut, grilled (broiled)	**231**	1 piece of fillet	42	0	7	0
Halibut, poached or steamed	**229**	1 piece of fillet	42	0	7	0
Halloumi cheese	**98**	1 thick slice (⅛ block)	7	1	7	0
Halva	**265**	⅛ block	7	23	16	low
Ham, boiled	**167**	2 thick slices	29	0	5	0
Ham, canned	**60**	1 medium slice	9	0	2	0
Ham, ready-sliced, no added water	**37**	1 medium slice	6	trace	1	0
Ham, roast	**174**	2 thick slices	25	4	6	low
Ham and cheese quiche	**476**	1 slice	23	24	32	low
Ham and chopped pork loaf	**35**	1 slice	2	trace	3	low
Ham and mushroom pizza, deep-pan	**292**	1 slice	8	35	11	medium

Food	kCalories per portion	Portion size	Protein g	Carbo-hydrate g	Fat g	Fibre
Ham and mushroom pizza, thin-crust	242	1 slice	8	26	9	medium
Ham and pineapple pizza, deep-pan	276	1 slice	8	31	11	medium
Ham and pineapple pizza, thin-crust	226	1 slice	8	22	9	medium
Ham and tomato quiche	479	1 slice	23	25	32	low
Ham sandwiches	341	1 round	11	34	18	medium
Hamburger, retail	253	1 burger in a bun	13	33	8	medium
Hamburger, home-made	437	1 thick burger in a bun	31	25	14	low
Hare, jugged	420	1 serving	30	7	30	low
Hare, roast	193	1 serving	30	0	9	0
Hare, stewed	192	1 serving	30	0	8	0
Haricot (navy) beans, canned, drained	92	3 heaped tablespoons	7	17	trace	high
Haricot beans, dried, soaked and cooked	95	3 heaped tablespoons	7	17	trace	high
Haricot mutton/lamb	252	1 serving	21	24	9	medium
Harusami noodles	251	1 serving	2	57	trace	low
Hash browns	138	1 serving	1	16	8	medium
Haslet	30	1 slice	2	2	2	low
Havarti cheese	100	1 slice	6	0	9	0
Hawaiian pizza, deep-pan	276	1 slice	8	31	11	medium

Food	kCalories per portion	Portion size	Protein g	Carbo- hydrate g	Fat g	Fibre
Hawaiian pizza, thin-crust	226	1 slice	8	22	9	medium
Hazelnut (filbert) ice cream	91	1 scoop	2	12	4	low
Hazelnuts, shelled	162	25 g/1 oz/¼ cup	3	1	16	high
Hearts, braised	190	1 serving	33	8	8	high
Hearts, roast, stuffed	295	1 serving	27	4	19	low
Hearts, stewed	179	1 serving	31	0	6	0
Herring, grilled (broiled)	202	1 medium fish	21	0	13	0
Herring, filleted, fried (sautéed), in oatmeal	351	1 medium fish	34	2	22	low
Herring, pickled	39	1 small fillet	2	1	3	0
Herring, rollmop	180	1 roll	12	6	12	0
Herring, soused	180	1 roll	12	6	12	0
Herring roes, fried (sautéed)	244	1 serving	21	5	16	low
Herring roes, on toast	399	1 serving plus 1 slice of toast	24	23	25	low
Hobnobs	69	1 biscuit (cookie)	1	9	3	low
Hobnobs, chocolate	96	1 biscuit	1	12	5	low
Hobnob creams, chocolate or vanilla	63	1 biscuit	1	8	3	low
Hoisin sauce	27	1 tablespoon	trace	6	trace	low
Hollandaise sauce	214	3 tablespoons	8	trace	25	0
Homewheat biscuits (cookies), chocolate	87	1 biscuit	1	11	4	low

Food	kCalories per portion	Portion size	Protein g	Carbo-hydrate g	Fat g	Fibre
Homewheat biscuits, chocolate, mini	18	1 biscuit	trace	2	1	low
Honey	43	1 tablespoon	trace	13	0	0
Honey cake	89	1 slice	trace	14	0	low
Honey crispix, dry	95	25 g/1 oz/½ cup	1	21	trace	low
Honey crispix, with semi-skimmed milk	209	5 heaped tablespoons	6	33	3	low
Honey crispix, with skimmed milk	193	5 heaped tablespoons	6	33	1	low
Honey loops, dry	92	25 g/1 oz/½ cup	2	19	1	medium
Honey loops, with semi-skimmed milk	205	5 heaped tablespoons	7	37	3	medium
Honey loops, with skimmed milk	189	5 heaped tablespoons	7	37	1	medium
Honey mustard	7	1 teaspoon	trace	trace	trace	0
Honey nut cheerios, dry	93	25 g/1 oz/½ cup	2	20	1	medium
Honey nut cheerios, with semi-skimmed milk	172	5 heaped tablespoons	6	30	3	medium
Honey nut cheerios, with skimmed milk	156	5 heaped tablespoons	6	30	1	medium
Honey nut corn flakes, dry	97	25 g/1 oz/½ cup	2	20	1	low
Honey nut corn flakes, with semi-skimmed milk	213	5 heaped tablespoons	7	39	3	low

Food	kCalories per portion	Portion size	Protein g	Carbo-hydrate g	Fat g	Fibre
Honey nut corn flakes, with skimmed milk	197	5 heaped tablespoons	7	39	1	low
Honey nut shredded wheat, dry	95	25 g/1 oz/½ cup	3	17	2	high
Honey nut shredded wheat, with semi-skimmed milk	210	3 heaped tablespoons	8	34	5	high
Honey nut shredded wheat, with skimmed milk	194	3 heaped tablespoons	8	34	3	high
Honey rice krispies, dry	35	25 g/1 oz/½ cup	1	22	trace	low
Honey rice krispies, with semi-skimmed milk	209	5 heaped tablespoons	6	42	2	low
Honey rice krispies, with skimmed milk	193	5 heaped tablespoons	6	42	trace	low
Honeycomb	42	1 tablespoon	trace	11	1	0
Honeydew melon	63	1 large wedge	1	15	trace	medium
Horlicks, made with semi-skimmed milk	202	1 mug	11	32	5	low
Horlicks, made with skimmed milk	170	1 mug	11	32	1	low
Horlicks, instant, chocolate, made with water	128	1 mug	5	21	3	medium
Horlicks, instant, chocolate malted, made with water	129	1 mug	3	24	2	medium
Horlicks, instant, low-fat, made with water	127	1 mug	6	25	1	low

Food	kCalories per portion	Portion size	Protein g	Carbo-hydrate g	Fat g	Fibre
Horn of plenty mushrooms, fried (sautéed)	78	2 tablespoons	1	trace	8	low
Horn of plenty mushrooms, stewed	6	2 tablespoons	1	trace	trace	low
Horseradish, cream	11	1 teaspoon	trace	1	1	low
Horseradish, fresh, grated	24	1 tablespoon	trace	1	1	low
Horseradish, relish	5	1 teaspoon	trace	trace	trace	low
Horseradish, sauce	8	1 teaspoon	trace	1	trace	low
Hot and sour soup	129	2 ladlefuls	12	8	6	low
Hot chocolate See Drinking (sweetened) chocolate						
Hot cross bun	148	1 bun	4	26	4	medium
Hot cross bun, with butter	222	1 bun	4	26	12	medium
Hot cross bun, with low-fat spread	187	1 bun	4	26	8	medium
Hot dog	189	1 sausage plus 1 bun	7	22	9	medium
Hot dog, sausage only	82	1 sausage	3	1	7	low
Hot dog, with onions	230	1 sausage plus 1 bun	4	4	10	medium
Hot fudge sundae	180	1 sundae	3	30	5	0
Hummus	280	2 tablespoons	10	13	22	high
Hula hoops See Potato hoops						
Hungarian goulash	406	1 serving	28	16	22	medium
Huss See Rock salmon						

Food	kCalories per portion	Portion size	Protein g	Carbo-hydrate g	Fat g	Fibre
Ice cream, dairy, flavoured	89	1 scoop	2	11	4	low
Ice cream, dairy, vanilla	97	1 scoop	2	12	5	low
Ice cream, low-calorie, flavoured	67	1 scoop	2	8	3	low
Ice cream, low-calorie, vanilla	71	1 scoop	1	9	3	low
Ice cream, mixed, multi-flavours	91	1 scoop	2	12	4	low
Ice cream, non-dairy, flavoured	83	1 scoop	1	11	4	low
Ice cream, non-dairy, vanilla	89	1 scoop	2	11	4	low
Ice cream 99, with flake bar	175	1 cornet	5	31	13	low
Ice cream bombe	283	1 serving	4	18	17	0
Ice cream cone, double	222	2 scoops	5	34	8	low
Ice cream cone, single	131	1 scoop	3	22	4	low
Ice cream gâteau	227	1 slice	3	23	14	low
Ice lolly, any flavour	28	1 lolly	trace	7	trace	0
Ice pop, large	63	1 lolly	0	17	0	0
Ice pop, small	42	1 lolly	0	11	0	0
Ice split, any flavour	83 (average)	1 lolly	1	13	3	0
Iceberg lettuce	2	1 good handful	trace	1	0	low
Iced coffee	133	1 tumbler	6	10	8	0
Iced coffee, with sugar	173	1 tumbler	6	15	8	0

Food	kCalories per portion	Portion size	Protein g	Carbo-hydrate g	Fat g	Fibre
Iced (frosted) fancies	150	1 cake	1	25	5	low
Iced gems	117	1 small bag	2	25	1	low
Iced tea, with sugar	89	1 tumbler	0	20	0	0
Icing (frosting) *See individual types and flavours, e.g. Fondant icing, Chocolate fudge icing*						
Instant whipped dessert, made with semi-skimmed milk	103	1 serving	3	14	6	low
Instant whipped dessert, made with skimmed milk	88	1 serving	3	14	3	low
Instant whipped dessert, sugar-free, made with semi-skimmed milk	103	1 serving	3	11	7	0
Instant whipped dessert, sugar-free, made with skimmed milk	88	1 serving	3	11	6	0
Irish coffee	218	1 wine glass	1	7	14	0
Irish cream liqueur	102	1 single measure	1	6	5	0
Irish stew	336	1 serving	14	25	21	medium
Irn-bru	65	1 tumbler	0	21	trace	low
Irn-bru, diet	8	1 tumbler	0	2	trace	low
Isotonic drink	92	1 can/carton	trace	21	0	0
Italian pork sausage	216	1 sausage	13	1	17	0

Food	kCalories per portion	Portion size	Protein g	Carbo-hydrate g	Fat g	Fibre
Jacket potato See *also* Potato, baked	**272**	1 large potato	8	64	trace	high
Jaffa cake	**48**	1 individual cake	1	9	1	low
Jaffa cake, mini	**26**	1 small cake	trace	5	1	low
Jaffa cake muffin	**416**	1 bar	4	57	19	low
Jalousie, jam (conserve)	**319**	1 slice	3	33	20	low
Jalousie, mincemeat	**321**	1 slice	4	33	21	medium
Jam (conserve), any flavour	**39**	1 tablespoon	trace	10	0	0
Jam, any flavour, reduced-sugar	**18**	1 tablespoon	trace	5	trace	0
Jam (jelly) roll, steamed or baked	**391**	1 slice	5	52	19	medium
Jam ring biscuits (cookies)	**60**	1 biscuit	1	9	2	low
Jam sandwich cake	**302**	1 slice	4	64	5	low
Jam sandwich creams	**74**	1 biscuit (cookie)	1	9	3	low
Jam sponge cake	**302**	1 slice	4	64	5	low
Jam tart	**130**	1 individual tart	1	20	5	low
Jambalaya	**468**	1 serving	41	61	6	high
Japanese miso soup	**78**	2 ladlefuls	5	8	4	medium
Jarlsberg cheese	**105**	1 small wedge	7	1	8	0
Jellied consommé	**32**	2 ladlefuls	5	2	trace	0
Jellied eels	**70**	1 small serving	6	trace	6	0
Jello See Jelly						

Food	kCalories per portion	Portion size	Protein g	Carbo-hydrate g	Fat g	Fibre
Jelly (jello), any flavour	**91**	1 serving	2	22	0	0
Jelly, milk, made with semi-skimmed milk	**148**	1 serving	6	28	2	0
Jelly, milk, made with skimmed milk	**132**	1 serving	6	28	trace	0
Jelly, sugar-free, made up	**8**	1 serving	1	trace	trace	0
Jelly, yoghurt	**60**	1 serving	5	12	1	0
Jelly babies	**15**	1 sweet (candy)	trace	3	0	0
Jelly beans	**11**	1 bean	trace	3	0	0
Jelly roll See Jam roll *and* Swiss roll						
Jelly tots	**147**	1 small packet	trace	37	0	0
Jerk chicken	**256**	1 serving	32	15	8	high
Jerusalem artichokes, steamed or boiled	**41**	3 heaped tablespoons	2	11	0	high
Jugged hare	**420**	1 serving	30	7	30	low
Jumbo shrimp See King prawn						
Junket, made with semi-skimmed milk	**120**	1 serving	4	16	4	0
Junket, made with skimmed milk	**101**	1 serving	4	16	2	0
Just right, dry	**90**	25 g/1 oz/½ cup	2	19	1	medium

Food	kCalories per portion	Portion size	Protein g	Carbo-hydrate g	Fat g	Fibre
Just right, with semi-skimmed milk	**201**	5 heaped tablespoons	7	37	3	medium
Just right, with skimmed milk	**185**	5 heaped tablespoons	7	37	1	medium

Food	kCalories per portion	Portion size	Protein g	Carbo-hydrate g	Fat g	Fibre
Kalamares, fried (sautéed), in batter	**235**	1 serving	14	19	12	low
Kale, steamed or boiled	**24**	3 heaped tablespoons	2	1	1	medium
Kateifi	**322**	1 pastry	5	40	17	medium
Kedgeree, made with smoked fish	**498**	1 serving	43	31	24	low
Kedgeree, made with white fish	**495**	1 serving	44	31	24	low
Kelp	**4**	2 tablespoons	trace	1	trace	low
Kentucky fried chicken	**390**	2 pieces	29	10	27	low
Ketchup (catsup)	**15**	1 tablespoon	trace	4	trace	low
Kettle chips, all flavours	**136** (average)	1 good handful	1	12	9	medium
Kidney beans See Red kidney beans						
Kidneys, devilled	**158**	1 serving	21	2	7	0
Kidneys, lambs', fried (sautéed)	**155**	2 kidneys	25	0	6	0
Kidneys, lambs', grilled (broiled)	**109**	2 kidneys	26	0	4	0
Kidneys, ox, stewed	**172**	1 serving	26	0	8	0
Kidneys, pigs', fried (sautéed)	**155**	1 kidney	25	0	6	0
Kidneys, pigs', stewed	**153**	1 kidney	24	0	6	0
Kidneys turbigo	**363**	1 serving	48	2	54	low

Food	kCalories per portion	Portion size	Protein g	Carbo-hydrate g	Fat g	Fibre
Kielbasa sausage, grilled (broiled)	**81**	1 slice	3	1	7	0
King cone	**186**	1 cone	2	29	7	low
King prawn (jumbo shrimp)	**10**	1 prawn	2	0	trace	0
King prawn, battered	**45**	1 prawn	2	3	2	low
King prawn, in garlic butter	**48**	1 prawn	2	trace	2	low
King prawn masala	**164**	1 serving	24	5	6	low
Kipper, grilled (broiled)	**166**	1 medium fish	21	0	9	0
Kipper, poached or jugged	**166**	1 medium fish	21	0	9	0
Kipper fillets, boil-in-the-bag	**201**	1 fillet	16	0	15	0
Kipper fillets, canned in oil, drained	**140**	1 fillet	11	trace	12	0
Kipper pâté	**190**	1 serving	8	trace	17	0
Kir	**131**	1 wine glass	trace	8	0	0
Kirsch	**50**	1 single measure	trace	trace	0	0
Kit kat chocolate bar	**107**	2 fingers	1	13	5	low
Kit kat chocolate bar, chunky	**282**	1 bar	4	33	15	low
Kiwi fruit	**46**	1 fruit	1	11	trace	medium
Kleftiko (Greek slow-roast lamb with potatoes)	**741**	1 serving	67	11	49	medium
Knackwurst/knockwurst	**209**	1 sausage	8	1	19	0
Knickerbocker glory	**273**	1 tall glass	8	41	10	low
Kohlrabi, steamed or boiled	**36**	3 heaped tablespoons	1	5	0	medium

Food	kCalories per portion	Portion size	Protein g	Carbo-hydrate g	Fat g	Fibre
Krackawheat	**38**	1 cracker	1	5	2	low
Krispen, all flavours	**15** (average)	1 cracker	trace	3	trace	low
Kulfi ice cream	**340**	1 serving	4	9	32	low
Kumquat	**12**	1 fruit	0	3	0	low

Ladies' fingers

Food	kCalories per portion	Portion size	Protein g	Carbo-hydrate g	Fat g	Fibre
Ladies' fingers See Okra						
Lady fingers See Boudoir						
Lager	**87**	1 small	1	3	0	0
Lager, high-strength	226	1 small	1	7	0	0
Lager, low-alcohol	70	1 small	trace	4	0	0
Lamb, breast, roast	**410**	2 thick slices	19	0	37	0
Lamb, chop, lean, fried (sautéed)	277	1 chop	18	0	25	0
Lamb, chop, lean, grilled (broiled)	250	1 chop	18	0	23	0
Lamb, crown roast	488	1 serving	30	0	40	0
Lamb, cutlet, lean, fried	267	1 cutlet	15	0	22	0
Lamb, cutlet, lean, grilled	244	1 cutlet	15	0	20	0
Lamb, grillsteak, grilled	175	1 steak	14	1	13	0
Lamb, guard of honour	340	1 serving	25	10	22	low
Lamb, leg, roast, lean and fat	266	2 thick slices	26	0	18	0
Lamb, leg, roast, lean only	191	2 thick slices	29	0	8	0
Lamb, minced (ground), stewed	354	1 serving	39	0	22	0
Lamb, noisettes, fried	245	2 noisettes	28	0	14	0
Lamb, noisettes, grilled	222	2 noisettes	28	0	12	0
Lamb, shank, slow-roasted	465	1 shank	45	0	31	0

Food	kCalories per portion	Portion size	Protein g	Carbo-hydrate g	Fat g	Fibre
Lamb, shoulder, roast, lean and fat	316	3 medium slices	20	0	26	0
Lamb, shoulder, roast, lean only	196	3 medium slices	24	0	11	0
Lamb, steak, fried (sautéed)	357	1 steak	51	0	16	0
Lamb, steak, grilled (broiled)	334	1 steak	51	0	14	0
Lamb byriani	828	1 serving	22	75	51	medium
Lamb curry	935	1 serving	37	10	82	medium
Lamb curry, with rice	1183	1 serving	42	66	84	medium
Lamb goulash	446	1 serving	28	16	26	medium
Lamb kheema	656	1 serving	29	5	58	low
Lamb rogan josh	691	1 serving	51	17	41	medium
Lamb stew	369	1 serving	16	30	13	medium
Lamb tagine	724	1 serving	47	14	54	medium
Lambrusco	70	1 wine glass	trace	2	0	0
Lamingtons	233	1 individual cake	3	36	2	medium
Lancashire cheese	93	1 small wedge	58	trace	8	0
Lancashire hot-pot	342	1 serving	28	30	13	high
Langoustines	10	1 langoustine	2	0	trace	0
Langues de chat	28	1 biscuit (cookie)	trace	3	1	low
Lasagne, meat, home-made	650	1 serving	36	32	44	medium
Lasagne, meat, ready-prepared	306	1 serving	15	38	11	low

Food	kCalories per portion	Portion size	Protein g	Carbo-hydrate g	Fat g	Fibre
Lasagne, seafood	351	1 serving	22	32	16	high
Lasagne, vegetable	424	1 serving	15	50	10	high
Lassi	124	1 tumbler	6	26	trace	low
Leek	44	1 medium leek	4	6	1	high
Leek, roast	67	1 medium leek	1	3	3	high
Leek, sliced, steamed or boiled	21	3 heaped tablespoons	1	3	1	medium
Leek and potato soup, canned	94	2 ladlefuls	2	8	6	low
Leek and potato soup, home-made	117	2 ladlefuls	5	15	5	medium
Leek and potato soup, packet	80	2 ladlefuls	2	24	7	low
Leek vinaigrette	223	4 small leeks	1	3	23	medium
Leerdammer cheese	93	1 small wedge	7	trace	8	0
Lemon	12	1 fruit	trace	2	trace	0
Lemon and lime, sparkling	78	1 tumbler	trace	19	trace	0
Lemon and lime, sparkling, low-calorie	9	1 tumbler	trace	2	trace	0
Lemon barley water, diluted	40	1 tumbler	trace	9	trace	0
Lemon cake	384	1 slice	5	54	18	low
Lemon cheesecake	273	1 serving	5	30	13	low
Lemon chicken	356	1 serving	58	3	13	0
Lemon curd	42	1 tablespoon	trace	9	1	low
Lemon curd tart	150	1 individual tart	1	22	6	low

Food	kCalories per portion	Portion size	Protein g	Carbo-hydrate g	Fat g	Fibre
Lemon danish pastry	**263**	1 pastry	4	34	13	medium
Lemon drop cakes	**130**	1 individual cake	1	20	5	low
Lemon drop sweets (candies)	**20**	1 sweet	0	5	0	0
Lemon juice, pure	**1**	1 tablespoon	trace	trace	trace	low
Lemon meringue pie	**362**	1 slice	5	50	16	low
Lemon mousse	**227**	1 serving	4	38	8	low
Lemon puffs	**69**	1 biscuit (cookie)	1	7	4	low
Lemon sauce	**43**	2 tablespoons	trace	10	0	0
Lemon sherbert sweets (candies)	**20**	1 sweet	0	5	0	0
Lemon slice	**125**	1 cake	1	19	5	low
Lemon sole, fried (sautéed), in breadcrumbs	**342**	1 medium fish	25	15	21	low
Lemon sole, grilled (broiled)	**158**	1 medium fish	25	0	4	0
Lemon sole, poached or steamed	**128**	1 medium fish	29	0	1	0
Lemon sorbet	**65**	1 scoop	trace	17	trace	0
Lemon soufflé	**315**	1 serving	6	21	41	0
Lemon sponge pudding	**308**	1 serving	3	50	11	low
Lemon squash, diluted	**53**	1 tumbler	trace	13	trace	0
Lemon squash, low-calorie, diluted	**2**	1 tumbler	trace	trace	0	0
Lemon tango	**98**	1 tumbler	trace	23	trace	0

Food	kCalories per portion	Portion size	Protein g	Carbo-hydrate g	Fat g	Fibre
Lemon tango, low-calorie	8	1 tumbler	trace	trace	trace	0
Lemon tea, instant	88	1 cup	trace	22	0	0
Lemon tea, instant, low-calorie	5	1 cup	trace	1	trace	0
Lemon water ice	65	1 scoop	trace	17	trace	0
Lemonade, home-made	141	1 tumbler	trace	35	trace	0
Lemonade, sparkling	42	1 tumbler	trace	11	0	0
Lemonade, sparkling, low-calorie	1	1 tumbler	0	trace	0	0
Lemonade shandy	60	1 tumbler	0	14	trace	low
Lentil and bacon soup, canned	120	2 ladlefuls	4	15	2	medium
Lentil and bacon soup, home-made	302	2 ladlefuls	14	26	51	medium
Lentil and tomato soup, canned	108	2 ladlefuls	6	20	trace	medium
Lentil rissoles	90	1 rissole	7	15	3	high
Lentil soup, canned	92	2 ladlefuls	8	25	8	medium
Lentil soup, home-made	198	2 ladlefuls	9	26	8	medium
Lentil stew	282	1 serving	19	49	2	high
Lentils, green or brown, soaked and cooked	105	3 heaped tablespoons	9	17	1	high
Lentils, red, cooked	100	3 heaped tablespoons	8	17	trace	medium

Food	kCalories per portion	Portion size	Protein g	Carbo-hydrate g	Fat g	Fibre
Lettuce	2	1 good handful	trace	1	0	low
Lettuce soup, rich, home-made	127	2 ladefuls	2	19	3	low
Light corn syrup See Golden syrup						
Lilt, pineapple and grapefruit	90	1 tumbler	0	23	0	0
Lilt, pineapple and grapefruit, diet	8	1 tumbler	0	0	0	0
Lima beans See Butter beans						
Limburger cheese	93	1 small wedge	6	trace	8	0
Lime	9	1 fruit	trace	1	0	0
Lime cordial, diluted	36	1 tumbler	trace	10	trace	0
Lime pickle	23	1 tablespoon	trace	2	2	low
Lime squash, low-calorie, diluted	2	1 tumbler	trace	trace	0	0
Limeade	16	1 tumbler	trace	4	0	0
Limeade and lager	54	1 tumbler	trace	13	trace	0
Lincoln biscuits (cookies)	43	1 biscuit	trace	6	2	low
Lincolnshire sausage, grilled (broiled)	117	1 sausage	7	3	9	low
Ling, grilled (broiled)	168	1 piece of fillet	37	0	1	low
Linguine (pasta ribbons), dried, boiled	239	1 serving	8	51	2	medium

Food	kCalories per portion	Portion size	Protein g	Carbo-hydrate g	Fat g	Fibre
Linguine, fresh, boiled	301	1 serving	11	57	2	medium
Lion bar, chocolate	145	1 standard bar	1	20	6	low
Lion bar, ice cream	227	1 standard bar	3	24	13	low
Liqueur coffee	218	1 wine glass	1	7	14	0
Liquorice all-sorts	29	1 sweet (candy)	trace	7	trace	0
Liquorice caramels	39	1 sweet (candy)	trace	7	1	0
Liquorice sticks	5	1 stick	0	1	0	0
Liver, calves', braised	165	3 thin slices	22	3	7	low
Liver, calves', fried (sautéed), in seasoned flour	254	3 thin slices	27	7	13	0
Liver, lambs', fried (sautéed), in seasoned flour	232	3 thin slices	23	4	14	0
Liver, pigs', stewed	189	1 serving	26	4	8	0
Liver and bacon, fried (sautéed)	498	1 serving	43	8	46	0
Liver and onions, fried (sautéed)	396	1 serving	25	18	25	medium
Liver casserole	220	1 serving	31	2	9	low
Liver pâté	158	1 serving	6	trace	14	0
Liver pâté, en croûte	596	1 slice	16	24	49	low
Liver pâté, low-fat	131	1 serving	7	2	10	0
Liver pâté, with toast and butter	496	1 serving plus 2 slices of toast	13	35	31	medium

Food	kCalories per portion	Portion size	Protein g	Carbo-hydrate g	Fat g	Fibre
Liver sausage, sliced	57	1 slice	2	trace	5	0
Liver sausage, spreading	77	1 tablespoon	3	1	7	low
Livers, chicken, fried (sautéed)	194	1 serving	21	3	11	0
Lobster	126	½ medium lobster	24	0	4	0
Lobster bisque	108	2 ladlefuls	13	10	4	low
Lobster mayonnaise salad	363	½ medium lobster	26	5	28	high
Lobster newburg	225	1 serving	20	23	5	low
Lobster salad	157	½ medium lobster	26	5	5	high
Lobster tails, fried (sautéed), in breadcrumbs	316	1 serving	12	29	18	low
Lobster thermidor	376	½ medium lobster	33	7	19	0
Lockets	165	1 tube	0	41	0	0
Loganberries	55	3 heaped tablespoons	1	13	trace	medium
Loganberries, stewed	50	3 heaped tablespoons	trace	11	trace	medium
Loganberries, stewed with sugar	80	3 heaped tablespoons	trace	21	trace	medium
Loquats	7	1 fruit	trace	2	trace	low
Low-fat spread	117	25 g/1 oz/2 tbsp	3	trace	12	0
Low-fat spread	39	1 small knob	1	trace	4	0
Lucozade	137	1 tumbler	trace	36	0	0
Lumachi (pasta shapes), dried, boiled	198	1 serving	7	42	1	medium

Food	KCalories per portion	Portion size	Protein g	Carbo-hydrate g	Fat g	Fibre
Lumachi, fresh, boiled	235	1 serving	9	45	2	medium
Lumpfish roe	40	1 tablespoon	4	1	3	0
Lunch tongue	53	1 slice	4	trace	3	0
Luncheon meat	100	1 slice	4	1	9	0
Lychees	5	1 fruit	trace	1	trace	low
Lychees, canned in syrup	66	3 heaped tablespoons	trace	18	trace	low
Lymeswold cheese	106	1 small wedge	4	trace	10	0

Food	kCalories per portion	Portion size	Protein g	Carbo-hydrate g	Fat g	Fibre
M&Ms, chocolate	219	1 small bag	2	31	1	0
M&Ms, peanut	231	1 small bag	5	26	12	low
Macadamia nuts	112	1 small handful	1	1	12	high
Macaroni, dried, boiled	198	1 serving	7	42	1	medium
Macaroni, fresh, boiled	235	1 serving	9	45	1	medium
Macaroni cheese	436	1 serving	23	46	17	medium
Macaroni cheese, canned	188	1 small can	7	19	10	low
Macaroons, almond	120	1 macaroon	3	13	7	medium
Macaroons, coconut	117	1 macaroon	1	16	5	medium
Macedoine (mixed, diced vegetables), steamed or boiled	42	3 heaped tablespoons	3	7	trace	high
Mackerel, fried (sautéed)	310	1 medium fish	35	0	19	0
Mackerel, grilled (broiled)	279	1 medium fish	38	0	15	0
Mackerel, smoked	531	1 fillet	28	0	46	0
Mackerel, smoked pâté	599	1 serving	19	0	58	0
Mackerel, soused	165	1 roll	16	6	9	0
Madeira, dry	58	1 double measure	trace	trace	0	0
Madeira, sweet	68	1 double measure	trace	trace	0	0
Madeira cake	393	1 slice	5	58	17	low
Madelaines	137	1 cake	2	16	8	low
Magnum, all flavours	300 (average)	1 ice cream	4	27	20	0

Food	kCalories per portion	Portion size	Protein g	Carbo-hydrate g	Fat g	Fibre
Maids of honour	207	1 individual tart	2	35	12	low
Maître d'hôtel butter	92	1 tablespoon	trace	trace	10	0
Malt loaf	80	1 slice	2	17	1	low
Maltesers	183	1 small packet	3	18	5	0
Mandarin orange	30	1 fruit	1	7	trace	medium
Mandarin oranges, canned in natural juice	32	3 heaped tablespoons	1	8	trace	low
Mandarin oranges, canned in syrup	52	3 heaped tablespoons	trace	13	trace	low
Mangetout (snow peas)	16	3 heaped tablespoons	2	2	trace	medium
Mangetout, steamed or boiled	13	3 heaped tablespoons	1	2	trace	medium
Mangetout, stir-fried	35	3 heaped tablespoons	2	2	2	medium
Mango	97	1 medium fruit	1	24	trace	high
Mango, canned in syrup	77	3 heaped tablespoons	trace	20	trace	high
Mango chutney	43	1 tablespoon	trace	7	2	low
Mango mousse	137	1 serving	4	18	6	low
Mango sorbet	88	1 scoop	trace	24	trace	medium
Mangosteen	20	1 fruit	trace	5	trace	medium
Mangosteen, canned in syrup	73	3 heaped tablespoons	trace	18	trace	medium
Maple syrup	53	1 tablespoon	0	15	0	0
Maraschino cherries	12	1 fruit	trace	3	trace	low
Maraschino liqueur	64	1 single measure	trace	8	0	0

Food	kCalories per portion	Portion size	Protein g	Carbo-hydrate g	Fat g	Fibre
Marble cake	371	1 slice	5	55	14	medium
Marc	55	1 single measure	trace	trace	0	0
Margarine	185	25 g/1 oz/2 tbsp	trace	trace	20	0
Margarine	74	1 small knob	trace	trace	8	0
Margherita pizza, Italian-style	235	1 slice	9	25	12	medium
Marie biscuits (cookies)	35	1 biscuit	trace	6	1	low
Marlin steak, fried (sautéed)	294	1 steak	44	0	14	0
Marlin steak, grilled (broiled)	271	1 steak	44	0	9	0
Marmalade	39	1 tablespoon	trace	0	10	low
Marmalade, reduced-sugar	21	1 tablespoon	trace	trace	10	0
Marmalade pudding	340	1 serving	6	45	16	medium
Marmalade tart	285	1 slice	2	46	11	medium
Marmite	9	1 teaspoon	2	trace	trace	0
Marrow (squash), steamed or boiled	9	3 heaped tablespoons	trace	2	trace	low
Marrow, stuffed with meat	306	1 large slice	23	38	8	low
Marrowfat peas, canned	100	3 heaped tablespoons	7	17	1	high
Marrowfat peas, soaked and boiled	82	3 heaped tablespoons	6	18	1	high
Mars chocolate bar	294	1 standard bar	3	45	11	0
Mars ice cream	209	1 standard bar	3	22	12	0
Marsala	79	1 double measure	trace	6	0	0

Food	kCalories per portion	Portion size	Protein g	Carbo-hydrate g	Fat g	Fibre
Mascarpone cheese	64	1 tablespoon	trace	trace	7	0
Marshmallows	15	1 sweet (candy)	trace	4	0	0
Marshmallow chocolate tea cakes	73	1 cake	1	13	2	low
Martini, dry	59	1 double measure	trace	3	0	0
Martini, sweet	75	1 double measure	trace	8	0	0
Marzipan	101	25 g/1 oz	1	17	4	medium
Matchmakers	10	1 stick	trace	1	trace	0
Matzos	100	1 cracker	3	23	trace	medium
Mayonnaise	104	1 tablespoon	trace	trace	11	0
Mayonnaise, low-calorie	40	1 tablespoon	trace	1	4	0
Mcchicken sandwich	375	1 sandwich	16	39	17	high
Meat and potato pie	330	1 serving	24	25	19	medium
Meat cobbler	489	1 serving	32	40	28	high
Meat paste	35	1 tablespoon	1	2	3	low
Meat pie	460	1 individual pie	18	32	28	low
Meatballs, fried (sautéed)	246	4 meatballs	28	0	15	0
Meatballs, grilled (broiled)	218	4 meatballs	27	0	12	0
Meatballs in gravy, canned	208	½ large can	11	9	14	low
Meatballs in tomato sauce, canned	227	½ large can	8	33	7	medium
Meatballs with spaghetti	718	1 serving	36	80	31	medium

Food	kCalories per portion	Portion size	Protein g	Carbo-hydrate g	Fat g	Fibre
Meatloaf	**208**	1 thick slice	21	10	9	low
Meatloaf, with tomato sauce	370	2 slices	30	22	18	medium
Mediterranean vegetables, roasted	**80**	1 serving	1	10	5	high
Melba toast	53	1 slice	2	11	trace	low
Melon See individual varieties, e.g. Cantaloupe melon						
Melon cocktail	**48**	1 serving	1	12	trace	low
Melon with parma ham	105	1 slice of melon plus 2 slices of ham	9	15	1	low
Melton mowbray pork pie	**677**	1 standard pie	18	45	48	medium
Meringue	**95**	1 meringue	1	24	trace	0
Meringue, with cream	162	1 meringue	1	24	7	0
Meringue nest, with fresh fruit	**141**	1 meringue	3	32	1	medium
Milk loaf	**60**	1 medium slice	2	12	1	low
Milk powder, dried (non-fat dried milk)	**52**	1 tablespoon	5	8	trace	0
Milk, channel island	**234**	300 ml/½ pt/1¼ cups	11	14	15	0
Milk, condensed, skimmed, sweetened	**267**	100 ml/3½ fl oz/ scant ½ cup	10	60	trace	0
Milk, condensed, whole, sweetened	**333**	100 ml/3½ fl oz/ scant ½ cup	8	55	10	0

Food	kCalories per portion	Portion size	Protein g	Carbo-hydrate g	Fat g	Fibre
Milk, condensed, skimmed, unsweetened	**80**	100 ml/3½ fl oz/ scant ½ cup	10	11	trace	0
Milk, condensed, whole, unsweetened	**151**	100 ml/3½ fl oz/ scant ½ cup	8	8	9	0
Milk, semi-skimmed	**138**	300 ml/½ pt/1¼ cups	10	15	5	0
Milk, skimmed	**99**	300 ml/½ pt/1¼ cups	10	15	trace	0
Milk, whole	**198**	300 ml/½ pt/1¼ cups	10	14	12	0
Milk chocolate	**255**	1 standard bar	4	28	14	0
Milk classico ice lolly	**141**	1 lolly	2	9	13	0
Milk jelly (jello), made with semi-skimmed milk	**148**	1 serving	6	28	2	0
Milk jelly, made with skimmed milk	**132**	1 serving	6	28	trace	0
Milkshake, extra-thick	**238**	1 tumbler	6	42	5	low
Milkshake, made with granules and semi-skimmed milk	**138**	1 tumbler	6	23	3	low
Milkshake, made with granules and skimmed milk	**109**	1 tumbler	6	23	trace	low
Milkshake, made with syrup and semi-skimmed milk	**125**	1 tumbler	7	18	3	low
Milkshake, made with syrup and skimmed milk	**106**	1 tumbler	7	18	trace	low
Milk stick	**275**	1 lolly	3	24	18	0

Food	kCalories per portion	Portion size	Protein g	Carbo- hydrate g	Fat g	Fibre
Milky bar chocolate bar	163	1 standard bar	2	17	9	0
Milky way chocolate bar	117	1 standard bar	1	19	4	0
Milky way crispy rolls	131	1 roll	2	14	7	low
Millet flakes	80	25 g/1 oz/¼ cup	1	19	trace	medium
Mince *See individual meats*, e.g. Beef, minced						
Mince pie, sweet	244	1 individual pie	2	39	9	low
Mincemeat	41	1 tablespoon	trace	9	1	low
Minestrone, canned	85	2 ladlefuls	3	15	1	medium
Minestrone, home-made	248	2 ladlefuls	10	39	7	high
Minestrone, packet	79	2 ladlefuls	1	15	2	medium
Minibix with chocolate, dry	96	25 g/1 oz/½ cup	2	18	1	medium
Minibix with chocolate, with semi-skimmed milk	212	3 heaped tablespoons	7	35	4	medium
Minibix with chocolate, with skimmed milk	196	3 heaped tablespoons	7	35	3	medium
Minstrels	206	1 small packet	2	29	9	0
Mint chocolate chip ice cream	91	1 scoop	2	12	4	low
Mint imperials	18	1 sweet (candy)	0	5	0	0
Mint jelly (clear conserve)	38	1 tablespoon	trace	6	trace	0
Mint sauce	18	1 tablespoon	trace	4	trace	0
Miso soup, Japanese	78	1 serving	5	8	4	medium

Food	kCalories per portion	Portion size	Protein g	Carbo-hydrate g	Fat g	Fibre
Mississippi mud pie	**325**	1 slice	5	38	18	low
Mivi ice lolly, all flavours	**83** (average)	1 lolly	1	13	3	0
Mixed (candied) peel	**35**	1 tablespoon	trace	9	trace	low
Mixed salad	**31**	1 serving	2	5	1	high
Mixed salad, dressed	**128**	1 serving	2	5	18	high
Molasses	**38**	1 tablespoon	trace	10	0	0
Monkey nuts, raw, shelled See also Peanuts	**85**	1 small handful	4	2	7	high
Monkfish, grilled (broiled)	**170**	1 piece of fillet	31	0	3	0
Monkfish, roasted	**216**	1 piece of fillet	31	0	7	low
Monkfish stew	**330**	1 serving	30	43	5	medium
Monterey jack cheese	**106**	1 small wedge	7	trace	9	0
Morning rolls	**140**	1 roll	5	29	2	low
Mortadella	**47**	1 slice	2	trace	4	0
Moules à la crème	**372**	1 serving	21	11	21	low
Moules à la marinière	**238**	1 serving	21	11	7	low
Moussaka	**552**	1 serving	27	21	41	medium
Mozzarella cheese, danish	**77**	1 thick slice	6	trace	5	0
Mozzarella cheese, italian	**80**	¼ round cheese	5	1	6	0
Muesli, dry	**91**	25 g/1 oz/¼ cup	2	16	2	high
Muesli, with semi-skimmed milk	**203**	3 heaped tablespoons	8	33	5	high

Food	kCalories per portion	Portion size	Protein g	Carbo-hydrate g	Fat g	Fibre
Muesli, with skimmed milk	189	3 heaped tablespoons	8	33	3	high
Muffin, american	169	1 muffin	4	24	6	medium
Muffin, english	127	1 muffin	5	25	1	medium
Muffin, english, toasted, with butter	200	1 muffin	5	25	8	medium
Muffin, english, toasted, with low-fat spread	166	1 muffin	6	25	5	medium
Mulberries	43	3 heaped tablespoons	1	10	trace	medium
Mulled wine	105	1 wine glass	trace	5	0	0
Mullet, grey or red, grilled (broiled)	139	1 fillet	23	0	4	0
Mulligatawny soup, canned	137	2 ladlefuls	4	13	7	medium
Multi-grain start, dry	90	25 g/1 oz/½ cup	2	20	trace	medium
Multi-grain start, with semi-skimmed milk	201	5 heaped tablespoons	7	38	3	medium
Multi-grain start, with skimmed milk	185	5 heaped tablespoons	7	38	1	medium
Munchies	22	1 sweet	trace	3	1	0
Mung beans, dried, soaked and cooked	105	3 heaped tablespoons	7	18	trace	high
Mung beans, sprouted	6	1 good handful	trace	1	trace	high
Mung beans, sprouted, canned	12	3 heaped tablespoons	1	2	trace	high
Munster cheese	104	1 small wedge	7	trace	8	0

Food	kCalories per portion	Portion size	Protein g	Carbo-hydrate g	Fat g	Fibre
Muscatels, stoned (pitted)	41	1 small handful	trace	10	trace	low
Mushroom bhaji	123	1 bhaji	3	9	8	medium
Mushroom ketchup	6	1 teaspoon	trace	trace	trace	0
Mushroom omelette	295	2 eggs	14	trace	26	low
Mushroom pâté	117	½ small tub	3	4	9	0
Mushroom pâté, home-made	191	1 serving	1	1	19	low
Mushroom and cheese quiche	353	1 slice	14	18	26	low
Mushroom ragu	311	1 serving	4	3	30	low
Mushroom risotto	341	1 serving	5	52	14	low
Mushroom pasta sauce	45	¼ jar	trace	7	10	0
Mushroom sauce, made with semi-skimmed milk	99	5 tablespoons	3	8	6	low
Mushroom sauce, made with skimmed milk	89	5 tablespoons	3	8	5	low
Mushroom soup, cream of, canned	106	2 ladlefuls	2	8	8	0
Mushroom soup, home-made	156	2 ladlefuls	7	14	2	low
Mushroom soup, low-fat, canned	48	2 ladlefuls	2	7	1	low
Mushroom soup, packet	118	2 ladlefuls	4	21	2	0
Mushroom soup, instant	96	1 mug	trace	13	5	0

Food	kCalories per portion	Portion size	Protein g	Carbo-hydrate g	Fat g	Fibre
Mushrooms See also individual types, e.g. Shiitake mushrooms	2	1 medium mushroom	trace	trace	trace	low
Mushrooms, breaded	196	1 serving	3	8	16	medium
Mushrooms, button, sliced and fried (sautéed)	78	1 serving	1	trace	8	medium
Mushrooms, large, flat, fried	157	2 large mushrooms	2	trace	16	medium
Mushrooms, stewed	5	3 heaped tablespoons	1	trace	trace	medium
Mushrooms, stuffed	53	1 large mushroom	2	4	2	low
Mushrooms à la grecque	171	1 serving	2	4	30	low
Mushy peas, canned	69	3 heaped tablespoons	6	16	trace	high
Mussels, cooked, shelled	3	1 mussel	trace	trace	trace	0
Mussels, smoked, canned, drained	96	½ small can	2	2	5	0
See also Moules						
Mustard See individual varieties, e.g. Dijon mustard						
Mustard and cress	2	1 tablespoon	trace	trace	trace	medium
Mustard butter	118	1 tablespoon	trace	trace	6	0
Mustard chicken	176	1 breast	26	3	5	0
Mustard sauce, made with semi-skimmed milk	103	5 tablespoons	3	8	6	low
Mustard sauce, made with skimmed milk	93	5 tablespoons	3	8	5	low

Food	kCalories per portion	Portion size	Protein g	Carbo-hydrate g	Fat g	Fibre
Mutton, boiled	**253**	2 thick slices	28	0	16	0
Mutton, haricot	**252**	1 serving	21	24	9	medium
Mutton pie	**225**	1 individual pie	8	24	5	medium
Mutton stew	**369**	1 serving	14	24	21	medium

Food	kCalories per portion	Portion size	Protein g	Carbo-hydrate g	Fat g	Fibre
Naan bread, plain	175	1 small bread	6	29	4	medium
Nachos with cheese	346	6 pieces	9	36	19	low
Napoletana pizza	247	1 slice	10	25	13	medium
Napoletana sauce	61	¼ jar	2	9	2	low
Navy beans See Haricot beans						
Neapolitan ice cream	86	1 scoop	2	10	4	0
Nectarine	52	1 fruit	2	12	trace	medium
Nesquick cereal, dry	98	25 g/1 oz/½ cup	1	21	1	low
Nesquick cereal, with semi-skimmed milk	179	5 heaped tablespoons	5	31	3	low
Nesquick cereal, with skimmed milk	163	5 heaped tablespoons	5	31	1	low
Nesquick milk shake flavouring See Milkshakes						
Neufchatel cheese	74	1 small wedge	3	1	7	0
Nice biscuits (cookies)	35	1 biscuit	trace	5	1	low
Niçoise salad	308	1 serving	21	34	11	high
Noilly prat	59	1 double measure	trace	3	0	0
Noisettes of lamb, grilled (broiled)	222	2 noisettes	28	0	12	0
Noodles, dried, boiled	239	1 serving	8	51	2	medium

Food	kCalories per portion	Portion size	Protein g	Carbo-hydrate g	Fat g	Fibre
Noodles, fresh, boiled	301	1 serving	11	57	2	medium
See also individual types, e.g. Chinese egg noodles						
Norwegian apple cake	252	1 slice	3	32	10	high
Norwegian blue cheese	87	1 small wedge	5	trace	7	0
Norwegian cream	835	1 serving	6	25	79	0
Nut brittle	226	1 standard bar	3	34	9	medium
Nut cutlet	139	1 cutlet	5	5	10	medium
Nut rissole	203	1 rissole	7	6	18	medium
Nut roast	366	1 serving	12	13	29	high
Nutri-grain breakfast bars, all flavours	130 (average)	1 bar	1	24	3	medium
Nuts See individual varieties, e.g. brazil nuts						
Nuts, mixed	151	25 g/1 oz/¼ cup	6	2	13	high
Nuts and raisins	108	1 small handful	3	7	7	high

Food	kCalories per portion	Portion size	Protein g	Carbo-hydrate g	Fat g	Fibre
Oat bran	**51**	1 tablespoon	2	9	1	high
Oat bran crispbread	**27**	1 crispbread	1	5	trace	medium
Oat bran flakes, dry	**87**	25 g/1 oz/½ cup	2	16	1	high
Oat bran flakes, with semi-skimmed milk	**197**	5 heaped tablespoons	8	33	4	high
Oat bran flakes, with skimmed milk	**181**	5 heaped tablespoons	8	33	2	high
Oat cereal, instant See Ready brek						
Oat flakes, dry	**96**	25 g/1 oz/½ cup	3	17	18	high
Oat flakes, with semi-skimmed milk	**211**	5 heaped tablespoons	9	33	5	high
Oat flakes, with skimmed milk	**195**	5 heaped tablespoons	9	33	3	high
Oat krunchies, dry	**98**	25 g/1 oz/½ cup	2	19	1	medium
Oat krunchies, with semi-skimmed milk	**214**	5 heaped tablespoons	6	25	3	medium
Oat krunchies, with skimmed milk	**198**	5 heaped tablespoons	6	25	1	medium
Oatcakes	**59**	1 oatcake	1	8	2	medium
Oatmeal	**94**	25 g/1 oz/¼ cup	3	16	2	medium
Oatmeal porridge, made with semi-skimmed milk	**207**	1 serving	11	32	6	medium

Food	kCalories per portion	Portion size	Protein g	Carbo-hydrate g	Fat g	Fibre
Oatmeal porridge, made with skimmed milk	**191**	1 serving	11	32	6	medium
Oatmeal porridge, made with water	**150**	1 serving	4	26	4	medium
Oats, rolled	**100**	25 g/1 oz/¼ cup	3	18	1	medium
Oats, rolled, porridge, made with semi-skimmed milk	**217**	1 serving	9	35	6	medium
Oats, rolled, porridge, made with skimmed milk	**201**	1 serving	9	35	4	medium
Oats, rolled, porridge, made with water	**160**	1 serving	5	29	4	medium
Octopus	**164**	1 serving	30	4	2	0
Octopus, marinated in olive oil	**200**	½ small can	12	2	16	0
Ogen melon	**57**	½ melon	2	13	trace	medium
Oil, all types	**135**	1 tablespoon	trace	0	15	0
Okra (ladies' fingers), steamed or boiled	**28**	3 heaped tablespoons	2	3	1	high
Okra, stir-fried	**269**	3 heaped tablespoons	4	4	26	high
Olives, black or green	**7**	1 olive	trace	trace	1	medium
Olives, stuffed	**4**	1 olive	trace	trace	trace	medium
Olives, with feta cheese	**19**	1 piece of each	1	trace	2	low

Food	kCalories per portion	Portion size	Protein g	Carbo-hydrate g	Fat g	Fibre
Omelette See also individual fillings, e.g. Cheese omelette	256	2 eggs	14	trace	22	0
Omelette arnold bennet	373	2 eggs	25	trace	29	0
Onion	36	1 medium onion	1	8	trace	medium
Onion, fried (sautéed)	82	2 tablespoons	1	7	5	medium
Onion, pickled	4	1 onion	trace	1	trace	low
Onion, spring (scallion)	3	1 onion	trace	trace	trace	low
Onion, stuffed	190	1 large onion	13	19	8	high
Onion bhaji	123	1 bhaji	3	9	8	medium
Onion dip	27	2 tablespoons	4	1	1	0
Onion pakoras	148	1 pakora	3	9	11	medium
Onion rings, deep-fried in batter or breadcrumbs	97	5 rings	1	9	6	low
Onion sauce, made with semi-skimmed milk	64	5 tablespoons	2	6	4	low
Onion sauce, made with skimmed milk	55	5 tablespoons	2	6	3	low
Onion soup, cream of, canned	88	2 ladlefuls	1	8	6	low
Onion soup, french, home-made	94	2 ladlefuls	2	8	6	low
Onion soup, french, packet	104	2 ladlefuls	2	20	1	low

Food	kCalories per portion	Portion size	Protein g	Carbo-hydrate g	Fat g	Fibre
Onion soup, french, with cheese croûte	226	2 ladlefuls plus 1 croûte	9	21	8	low
Onion soup, white, home-made	121	2 ladlefuls	6	12	3	low
Onion soup, white, packet	77	2 ladlefuls	trace	4	trace	low
Onions in white sauce	36	3 heaped tablespoons	1	6	1	high
Orange	57	1 fruit	6	13	1	medium
Orange and pineapple pure fruit juice	84	1 tumbler	1	22	trace	0
Orange and pineapple squash, diluted	96	1 tumbler	trace	22	trace	0
Orange and pineapple squash, low-calorie, diluted	22	1 tumbler	trace	5	trace	0
Orange barley water, diluted	40	1 tumbler	trace	10	trace	0
Orange cake	290	1 slice	2	32	17	low
Orange curd	42	1 tablespoon	trace	9	1	low
Orange ice lolly	78	1 lolly	trace	19	0	0
Orange jelly (jello), fresh	40	1 serving	3	7	0	low
Orange mousse	137	1 serving	4	18	6	low
Orange pure fruit juice	72	1 tumbler	1	14	trace	low
Orange sauce	40	2 tablespoons	trace	10	trace	0
Orange squash, diluted	96	1 tumbler	trace	22	trace	0

Food	kCalories per portion	Portion size	Protein g	Carbo-hydrate g	Fat g	Fibre
Orange squash, low-calorie, diluted	24	1 tumbler	0	5	trace	0
Orange tango	92	1 tumbler	0	25	0	0
Orange tango, low-calorie	9	1 tumbler	trace	2	trace	0
Orange water ice	64	1 scoop	trace	16	0	0
Orangeade, sparkling	20	1 tumbler	0	4	0	0
Oranges in caramel	139	1 serving	6	33	1	medium
Original crunchy cereal, dry	97	25 g/1 oz/¼ cup	2	16	3	high
Original crunchy cereal, with semi-skimmed milk	250	3 heaped tablespoons	9	37	7	high
Original crunchy cereal, with skimmed milk	234	3 heaped tablespoons	9	37	5	high
Osso buco	382	1 serving	55	17	10	low
Ovaltine, made with semi-skimmed milk	197	1 mug	10	32	4	low
Ovaltine, made with skimmed milk	165	1 mug	10	32	trace	low
Ovaltine light, instant, made with water	72	1 mug	2	13	1	low
Oven chips (fries) See Chips						
Ox tongue, sliced	73	1 slice	5	0	6	0
Oxo	27	1 cube	2	4	trace	0
Oxo drink	10	1 mug	2	trace	0	0

Food	kCalories per portion	Portion size	Protein g	Carbo-hydrate g	Fat g	Fibre
Oxtail soup, canned	**88**	2 ladlefuls	5	10	3	0
Oxtail soup, packet	**54**	2 ladlefuls	3	8	2	0
Oxtail soup, instant	**77**	1 mug	1	14	2	0
Oxtail and vegetable stew	**318**	1 serving	38	7	15	high
Oyster mushrooms	**1**	1 mushroom	trace	trace	trace	low
Oyster mushrooms, fried (sautéed)	**77**	2 tablespoons	1	trace	8	low
Oyster mushrooms, stewed	**3**	2 tablespoons	1	trace	trace	low
Oysters	**7**	1 oyster	1	trace	trace	0
Oysters, fried (sautéed), in batter	**368**	6 oysters	12	40	18	low
Oysters, smoked, canned, drained	**103**	½ small can	9	trace	6	0

Food	kCalories per portion	Portion size	Protein g	Carbo-hydrate g	Fat g	Fibre
Paella, dried	**294**	1 serving	11	55	3	low
Paella, home-made	**411**	1 serving	40	34	11	low
Pain au chocolat	**236**	1 pastry	4	26	13	low
Pain au raisin	**212**	1 pastry	4	27	10	medium
Pain perdu	**213**	1 slice	6	17	18	low
Pak choi/soi	**19**	1 head	1	2	trace	medium
Pak choi/soi, steamed or boiled	**12**	3 heaped tablespoons	1	2	trace	medium
Pak choi/soi, stir-fried	**36**	3 heaped tablespoons	1	2	2	medium
Pakora	**148**	1 pakora	3	9	11	medium
Palm hearts, canned, drained	**9**	1 piece	1	2	trace	low
Palmiers	**83**	1 piece	1	12	6	low
Pancake, buckwheat	**45**	1 pancake	2	6	2	low
Pancake, potato	**207**	1 pancake	5	22	11	medium
Pancake, scotch	**44**	1 pancake	1	6	2	low
Pancake, wheat	**100**	1 pancake	2	8	6	low
See also Crêpe and Drop scone						
Pancake, with lemon and sugar	**120**	1 pancake	2	13	6	low
Pancake roll, large	**217**	1 large roll	7	21	12	low
Pancake roll, small	**70**	1 small roll	3	7	3	low
Pancetta, diced, fried (sautéed)	**248**	2 tablespoons	11	0	22	0

Food	kCalories per portion	Portion size	Protein g	Carbo-hydrate g	Fat g	Fibre
Panna cotta	328	1 serving	2	38	17	low
Pappardelle (pasta ribbons), dried, boiled	239	1 serving	8	51	2	medium
Pappardelle, fresh, boiled	301	1 serving	11	57	2	medium
Papaya	118	1 fruit	2	30	trace	high
Papaya, canned in natural juice	65	3 heaped tablespoons	trace	17	trace	low
Paratha	450	1 paratha	12	62	20	high
Parkin	185	1 piece	2	29	7	low
Parma ham	21	1 slice	4	0	1	0
Parma ham, with figs	87	1 fig plus 2 slices of ham	9	11	2	medium
Parma ham, with melon	105	1 slice of melon plus 2 slices of ham	9	15	1	low
Parmesan cheese	113	1 small chunk	10	trace	8	0
Parmesan cheese, grated	68	1 tablespoon	6	trace	5	0
Parsley sauce, made with semi-skimmed milk	99	5 tablespoons	3	8	6	low
Parsley sauce, made with skimmed milk	89	5 tablespoons	3	8	5	low
Parsnips	112	1 medium parsnip	3	22	2	high
Parsnips, roasted	156	4 pieces	3	22	6	high
Parsnips, steamed or boiled	66	1 serving	2	13	1	high

Food	kCalories per portion	Portion size	Protein g	Carbo- hydrate g	Fat g	Fibre
Partridge, roast	**212**	½ small bird	37	0	7	0
Passata (sieved tomatoes)	**29**	5 tablespoons	1	6	trace	0
Passion fruit	**17**	1 fruit	trace	4	trace	medium
Passion fruit ice cream	**83**	1 scoop	1	11	3	0
Pasta salad	**197**	1 serving	5	28	8	high
Pasta sauce, traditional, ready-made *See also individual flavours, e.g. Tomato and herb*	**58**	¼ jar	3	8	2	0
Pasta, shapes, dried, boiled	**198**	1 serving	7	42	1	medium
Pasta shapes, fresh, boiled	**235**	1 serving	9	45	2	medium
Pasta shapes, wholemeal, dried, boiled	**218**	1 serving	10	44	2	high
Pasta strands, all sizes, dried, boiled	**239**	1 serving	8	51	2	medium
Pasta strands, fresh, boiled	**301**	1 serving	11	57	2	medium
Pasta strands, wholemeal, dried, boiled	**259**	1 serving	31	152	6	high
Pastis	**61**	1 single measure	trace	trace	0	0
Pastrami	**99**	1 slice	5	1	8	0
Pastrami, on rye bread	**154**	1 slice of each	7	12	8	medium
Pâté, with toast and butter	**496**	1 serving plus 2 slices of toast	13	35	31	medium

Food	kCalories per portion	Portion size	Protein g	Carbo-hydrate g	Fat g	Fibre
Pavlova, topped with cream and fruit	**320**	1 serving	5	45	14	medium
Paw paw	**118**	1 fruit	2	30	trace	high
Pea and ham soup, canned	**150**	2 ladlefuls	6	19	6	high
Pea and ham soup, packet	**150**	2 ladlefuls	3	18	7	medium
Pea soup, canned	**188**	2 ladlefuls	10	30	6	medium
Pea soup, instant	**95**	1 mug	2	16	2	medium
Peach	**42**	1 peach	1	11	trace	medium
Peach and apple pure fruit juice	**84**	1 tumbler	1	20	trace	low
Peach melba	**169**	1 serving	3	28	5	medium
Peach pie	**261**	1 slice	2	38	12	low
Peach chutney	**24**	1 tablespoon	trace	6	trace	low
Peach squash, diluted	**96**	1 tumbler	trace	22	trace	0
Peach squash, low-calorie, diluted	**24**	1 tumbler	0	5	trace	0
Peaches, dried	**31**	1 piece	trace	8	trace	high
Peaches, dried, stewed with sugar	**103**	3 heaped tablespoons	1	27	trace	high
Peaches, dried, stewed	**77**	3 heaped tablespoons	1	20	trace	high
Peaches, sliced, canned in natural juice	**39**	3 heaped tablespoons	1	10	trace	low

Food	kCalories per portion	Portion size	Protein g	Carbo- hydrate g	Fat g	Fibre
Peaches, sliced, canned in syrup	55	3 heaped tablespoons	trace	14	trace	low
Peaches, whole, poached in natural juice	80	1 peach	1	16	trace	medium
Peaches, whole, poached in syrup	101	1 peach	1	16	trace	medium
Peaches, whole, poached in wine	136	1 peach	1	17	trace	medium
Peanut brittle	226	1 standard bar	3	34	9	medium
Peanut butter	93	1 tablespoon	3	2	8	high
Peanut butter and chocolate spread	89	1 tablespoon	2	5	7	medium
Peanut cookies	116	1 cookie	2	13	6	high
Peanut sauce	220	5 tablespoons	8	8	18	medium
Peanuts, dry-roasted	88	1 small handful	4	1	7	medium
Peanuts, raw, shelled	141	25 g/1 oz/¼ cup	6	3	11	medium
Peanuts, roasted, salted	90	1 small handful	4	1	8	medium
Peanuts and raisins	70	1 small handful	3	5	5	medium
Pear	45	1 fruit, unpeeled	trace	11	trace	high
Pear and apple pure fruit juice	78	1 tumbler	0	20	0	0
Pear condé	356	1 serving	4	51	15	medium
Pear drops	16	1 sweet (candy)	0	4	0	0

Food	kCalories per portion	Portion size	Protein g	Carbo-hydrate g	Fat g	Fibre
Pear melba	**179**	1 serving	2	32	5	low
Pears, canned in natural juice	**70**	2 halves	trace	17	trace	medium
Pears, canned in syrup	**100**	2 halves	trace	25	trace	medium
Pears, dried	**47**	1 piece	trace	12	trace	high
Pears, dried, stewed	**127**	3 heaped tablespoons	1	34	trace	high
Pears, dried, stewed with sugar	**140**	3 heaped tablespoons	1	37	trace	high
Pears, poached in wine	**139**	1 pear	1	7	trace	medium
Pears with chocolate sauce	**348**	1 serving	3	87	2	high
Peas, dried, soaked and boiled	**109**	3 heaped tablespoons	7	20	1	high
Peas, fresh, shelled	**83**	3 heaped tablespoons	7	11	1	high
Peas, fresh, shelled, cooked	**79**	3 heaped tablespoons	7	10	2	high
Peas, frozen, cooked	**69**	3 heaped tablespoons	6	10	1	high
Peas, garden, canned, drained	**80**	3 heaped tablespoons	5	13	1	high
Peas, marrowfat, canned, drained	**100**	3 heaped tablespoons	7	17	1	high
Peas, marrowfat, soaked and cooked	**82**	3 heaped tablespoons	6	18	1	high
Peas, mushy, canned	**81**	3 heaped tablespoons	6	14	1	medium
Peas, processed, canned, drained	**99**	3 heaped tablespoons	7	17	1	high
Peas, split, soaked and boiled	**262**	3 heaped tablespoons	10	20	16	high
Peas, sugar snap	**57**	10 pods	5	8	1	high

Food	kCalories per portion	Portion size	Protein g	Carbo-hydrate g	Fat g	Fibre
Peas, sugar snap, steamed or boiled	52	3 heaped tablespoons	5	5	1	high
Pease pudding	109	3 heaped tablespoons	7	20	1	high
Pecan nuts, shelled	196	25 g/1 oz/¼ cup	3	4	20	high
Pecan pie	502	1 slice	6	64	27	medium
Pecorino cheese	113	1 small chunk	10	trace	8	0
Peking duck with pancakes	665	1 portion with 6 small pancakes	39	32	42	high
Penne rigate (pasta shapes), dried, boiled	198	1 serving	7	42	1	medium
Penne rigate, fresh, boiled	235	1 serving	9	45	2	medium
Penguin chocolate bars, all flavours	135 (average)	1 standard bar	1	17	7	low
Peperami	132	1 stick	5	trace	12	low
Peppermint cordial, diluted	36	1 tumbler	0	10	trace	0
Peppermints	18	1 mint	0	5	0	0
Peperoni	27	1 slice	1	trace	2	0
Peperoni pizza	255	1 slice	14	28	10	low
Pepper (bell), green	22	1 pepper	1	4	trace	medium
Pepper, green, roasted	45	1 pepper	1	4	5	medium
Pepper, green, stewed	27	1 pepper	1	4	1	medium
Pepper, orange/yellow	35	1 pepper	1	7	trace	medium
Pepper, orange/yellow, roasted	58	1 pepper	1	7	5	medium

Food	kCalories per portion	Portion size	Protein g	Carbo-hydrate g	Fat g	Fibre
Pepper, orange/yellow, stewed	**39**	1 pepper	2	7	1	medium
Pepper, red	**48**	1 pepper	1	10	1	medium
Pepper red, roasted	**71**	1 pepper	2	10	6	medium
Pepper red, stewed	**51**	1 pepper	2	10	1	medium
Pepper, stuffed with meat	**266**	1 pepper	23	27	8	medium
Pepper, stuffed with rice	**202**	1 pepper	7	36	5	high
Pepsi	**88**	1 tumbler	0	22	0	0
Pepsi, diet	**0**	1 tumbler	trace	trace	0	0
Pepsi max	**1**	1 tumbler	trace	trace	0	0
Pernod	**55**	1 single measure	trace	trace	0	0
Perry, sparkling	**70**	1 wineglass	trace	0	2	0
Persimmon	**32**	1 fruit	trace	8	trace	low
Pesto sauce	**64**	1 tablespoon	1	trace	7	low
Petit pois, cooked	**49**	3 heaped tablespoons	7	17	1	high
Petit suisse cheese	**23**	1 small pot	3	1	1	0
Petits fours	**23**	1 sweet (candy)	trace	3	1	low
Petticoat tails shortbread	**448**	1 segment	5	52	24	medium
Pheasant, roast	**536**	¼ bird	81	0	24	0
Pheasant à la normande	**675**	¼ bird	91	3	46	0
Pheasant casserole	**588**	¼ bird	85	20	30	low
Physalis	**3**	1 fruit	trace	trace	trace	low
Piccalilli	**13**	1 tablespoon	trace	3	trace	low

Food	kCalories per portion	Portion size	Protein g	Carbo-hydrate g	Fat g	Fibre
Pickle, sweet	20	1 tablespoon	trace	5	trace	low
Pickle, tomato	24	1 tablespoon	trace	6	trace	low
Pickled egg	84	1 egg	7	trace	6	0
Pickled onion, large	4	1 onion	trace	1	trace	low
Pickled onion, silverskin	2	1 onion	trace	trace	trace	low
Picnic chocolate bar	230	1 standard bar	4	29	11	medium
Pigeon, roast	303	½ large or 1 small bird	37	0	18	0
Pigeon casserole	333	½ large or 1 small bird	39	8	20	low
Pigeon pie	470	1 serving	40	21	28	medium
Pike, grilled (broiled)	175	1 piece of fillet	38	0	1	0
Pikelets	91	1 pikelet	3	19	trace	low
Pilaff	286	1 serving	7	45	9	medium
Pilau rice	212	1 serving	4	46	2	medium
Pilchards, in tomato sauce, canned	177	2 pilchards	26	3	7	low
Pimientos, canned, drained	21	1 pimiento	1	8	1	low
Pimms	146	1 tumbler	trace	11	0	0
Pina colada	252	1 cocktail	1	32	3	low
Pine nuts	172	25 g/1 oz/¼ cup	3	1	17	medium
Pineapple	41	1 slice	trace	10	trace	medium
Pineapple, chunks, canned in natural juice	47	3 heaped tablespoons	trace	12	trace	low

Food	kCalories per portion	Portion size	Protein g	Carbo-hydrate g	Fat g	Fibre
Pineapple, glacé (candied)	13	1 piece	trace	4	trace	low
Pineapple, with kirsch	132	2 slices	trace	29	trace	medium
Pineapple and grapefruit drink, sparkling	88	1 tumbler	trace	24	trace	0
Pineapple and grapefruit pure fruit juice	94	1 tumbler	0	24	0	low
Pineapple and grapefruit squash, diluted	24	1 tumbler	0	5	trace	0
Pineapple and grapefruit squash, low-calorie, diluted	96	1 tumbler	trace	22	trace	0
Pineapple flambé	122	1 slice	2	24	1	medium
Pineapple pure fruit juice	82	1 tumbler	1	21	trace	low
Pineapple sorbet	65	1 scoop	trace	17	trace	0
Pineapple upside-down pudding	367	1 slice	4	58	14	medium
Pineapple water ice	65	1 scoop	trace	17	trace	0
Pink champagne	114	1 wineglass	trace	2	0	0
Pink gin	56	1 cocktail	trace	0	trace	0
Pink grapefruit	48	1 fruit	2	12	trace	medium
Pink grapefruit, with sugar	64	½ fruit	1	16	trace	medium
Pink grapefruit, with sugar, grilled (broiled)	64	½ fruit	1	16	trace	medium
Pinto beans, refried	107	3 heaped tablespoons	6	15	1	high

Food	kCalories per portion	Portion size	Protein g	Carbo-hydrate g	Fat g	Fibre
Pinto beans, soaked and boiled	137	3 heaped tablespoons	9	24	1	high
Piperade	260	1 serving	10	18	17	medium
Pistachio nut ice cream	91	1 scoop	2	12	4	low
Pistachio nuts, unshelled	50	1 small handful	1	1	4	high
Pitta bread, party size	16	1 tiny bread	1	4	trace	low
Pitta bread, white	160	1 bread	6	36	trace	medium
Pitta bread, white, small	80	1 small bread	3	18	trace	low
Pitta bread, wholemeal	137	1 bread	4	27	1	high
Pizza, cheese and tomato, deep-pan	300	1 slice	15	30	14	medium
Pizza, cheese and tomato, thin-crust *See also other flavours, e.g Ham and mushroom pizza*	235	1 slice	9	25	12	medium
Plaice, grilled (broiled)	202	1 medium fish	23	0	7	0
Plaice, fillet, fried (sautéed), in batter	488	1 fillet	28	24	31	low
Plaice, fillet, fried (sautéed), in breadcrumbs,	399	1 fillet	31	15	24	low
Plaice, fillet, steamed or poached	162	1 fillet	33	0	3	0
Plantain, boiled or steamed	112	½ plantain	1	28	trace	medium
Plantain, fried (sautéed)	267	½ plantain	1	47	9	medium

Food	kCalories per portion	Portion size	Protein g	Carbo-hydrate g	Fat g	Fibre
Ploughman's lunch	**650**	1 serving	22	54	36	medium
Plum, large	**30**	1 fruit	trace	7	trace	medium
Plum, small	**11**	1 fruit	trace	2	trace	medium
Plum crumble	**298**	1 serving	3	51	10	medium
Plum fool	**227**	1 serving	5	36	8	medium
Plum jam (conserve)	**39**	1 tablespoon	0	10	0	low
Plum pie	**290**	1 slice	3	14	39	medium
Plum pudding	**291**	1 serving	5	49	10	medium
Plum sauce, oriental	**27**	1 tablespoon	trace	6	trace	low
Plums, canned in syrup	**59**	3 heaped tablespoons	trace	15	trace	low
Plums, stewed	**27**	3 heaped tablespoons	1	6	trace	medium
Plums, stewed with sugar	**107**	3 heaped tablespoons	1	19	trace	medium
Poires belle hélène	**348**	1 serving	3	87	2	high
Polenta (cornmeal)	**214**	1 serving	5	46	1	low
Polenta, with cheese	**320**	1 serving	9	46	14	low
Polenta, with meat sauce	**431**	1 serving	17	51	18	low
Pollack, baked	**178**	1 piece of fillet	38	0	2	0
Polish pork sausage	**185**	¼ ring	8	1	16	0
Polo mints	**120**	1 tube	0	34	trace	0
Polo mints, sugar-free	**80**	1 tube	0	33	0	0
Polony	**70**	1 slice	2	3	5	0
Pomegranate	**51**	1 fruit	trace	12	trace	high

Food	kCalories per portion	Portion size	Protein g	Carbo-hydrate g	Fat g	Fibre
Pommes dauphinoise	**235**	1 serving	14	12	15	medium
Pompano, grilled (broiled)	**186**	1 piece of fillet	21	0	11	0
Pont l'évêque cheese	**101**	1 small wedge	6	trace	8	0
Pontefract cakes	**8**	1 sweet (candy)	0	2	0	0
Pop tarts, all flavours	**202** (average)	1 tart	3	36	6	medium
Poppadoms, fried (sautéed)	**48**	1 poppadom	3	6	2	low
Poppadoms, grilled (broiled)	**35**	1 poppadom	3	6	trace	low
Popcorn	**137**	1 small handful	trace	25	4	low
Popcorn, buttered	**72**	1 small handful	trace	12	3	low
Pork, chop, barbecued	**210**	1 chop	28	1	9	0
Pork, chop, lean, fried (sautéed)	**222**	1 chop	28	0	14	0
Pork, chop, lean, grilled (broiled)	**199**	1 chop	28	0	9	0
Pork, escalope, fried (sautéed)	**185**	1 escalope	31	0	7	0
Pork, loin, smoked	**56**	1 slice	8	0	3	0
Pork, minced (ground), lean, stewed	**147**	1 serving	21	0	7	0
Pork, roast, with crackling	**286**	2 thick slices	27	0	20	0
Pork, roast, without crackling	**185**	2 thick slices	31	0	7	0
Pork, sweet and sour	**303**	1 serving	26	31	9	medium

Food	kCalories per portion	Portion size	Protein g	Carbo-hydrate g	Fat g	Fibre
Pork and beef sausages, thick, fried (sautéed)	115	1 sausage	5	5	8	low
Pork and beef sausages, thick, grilled (broiled)	111	1 sausage	6	5	8	low
Pork and beef sausages, thin, fried	57	1 sausage	2	2	4	low
Pork and beef sausages, thin, grilled	55	1 sausage	3	2	4	low
Pork and vegetable stir-fry	273	1 serving	25	18	10	high
Pork belly, grilled (broiled)	398	1 slice	21	0	35	0
Pork belly, pickled	280	1 slice	20	0	22	0
Pork chop suey	321	1 serving	23	34	9	medium
Pork chow mein	323	1 serving	29	34	8	high
Pork crackling	101	1 finger-sized piece	trace	0	13	0
Pork kebab, marinated and grilled (broiled)	227	1 kebab	22	12	10	0
Pork pie	677	1 individual pie	18	45	49	medium
Pork rillettes	115	2 tablespoons	5	0	10	0
Pork sausages, extra-lean, fried (sautéed)	92	1 sausage	6	4	5	low
Pork sausages, extra-lean, grilled (broiled)	84	1 sausage	6	4	5	low
Pork sausages, thick, fried	123	1 sausage	5	4	10	low
Pork sausages, thick, grilled	117	1 sausage	7	5	10	low

Food	kCalories per portion	Portion size	Protein g	Carbo-hydrate g	Fat g	Fibre
Pork sausages, thin, fried	61	1 sausage	3	2	5	low
Pork sausages, thin, grilled	58	1 sausage	3	2	5	low
Pork spare ribs, barbecued american-style	288	2 ribs	25	2	16	0
Pork spare ribs, chinese-style	310	2 ribs	25	13	17	low
Pork teriyaki	133	1 serving	18	2	5	low
Porridge, instant *See Ready brek*						
Porridge, made with semi-skimmed milk	217	1 serving	9	35	6	medium
Porridge, made with skimmed milk	201	1 serving	9	35	4	medium
Porridge, made with water	160	1 serving	5	29	4	medium
Port salut cheese	100	1 small wedge	7	trace	8	0
Port, ruby, tawny or white	78	1 double measure	trace	6	0	0
Pot au chocolat	136	1 individual pot	2	19	5	low
Pot au chocolat, with cream	270	1 individual pot	2	20	19	low
Pot noodle, all flavours	305 (average)	1 pot	9	42	10	low
Potato, baked in jacket	272	1 large potato	8	64	trace	high
Potato, baked in jacket, with butter	346	1 large potato	8	64	8	high
Potato cake	126	1 cake	2	16	5	low

Food	kCalories per portion	Portion size	Protein g	Carbo-hydrate g	Fat g	Fibre
Potato chips See Crisps						
Potato hoops, all flavours	**131** (average)	1 small packet	1	14	8	low
Potato pancake	**207**	1 pancake	5	22	11	medium
Potato salad, canned	**176**	3 heaped tablespoons	2	15	10	low
Potato salad, with French dressing	**217**	3 heaped tablespoons	3	27	11	medium
Potato salad, with mayonnaise, home-made	**200**	3 heaped tablespoons	3	17	12	medium
Potato waffle, cooked	**84**	1 waffle	1	13	3	low
Potato wedges	**205**	6 wedges	10	34	4	high
Potatoes, chipped (fries), home-made	**312**	1 serving	6	50	11	high
Potatoes, creamed	**104**	1 serving	2	15	4	medium
Potatoes, croquette, shallow-fried	**107**	1 croquette	2	11	6	medium
Potatoes, duchesse	**82**	1 piece	2	8	2	medium
Potatoes, mashed, instant	**57**	3 heaped tablespoons	1	13	trace	low
Potatoes, mashed, with butter or margarine	**104**	3 heaped tablespoons	2	15	4	medium
Potatoes, new, boiled or steamed	**75**	3 small potatoes	1	18	trace	medium
Potatoes, new, canned	**63**	3 small potatoes	1	15	trace	low
Potatoes, steamed	**72**	2 pieces	2	17	trace	medium

Food	kCalories per portion	Portion size	Protein g	Carbo-hydrate g	Fat g	Fibre
Potatoes, roast	149	2 pieces	3	26	4	medium
Potatoes, scalloped	86	1 serving	3	11	4	medium
Potted cheese	267	1 small pot	12	1	23	0
Potted prawns (shrimp)	358	1 small pot	16	0	32	0
Potted shrimps	324	1 small pot	10	0	31	0
Poussin (cornish hen), roast, with skin	668	1 bird	57	0	47	0
Poussin, roast, without skin	295	1 bird	51	0	8	0
Poussin, spatchcocked, grilled (broiled)	428	1 bird	36	0	30	0
Praline ice cream	91	1 scoop	2	12	4	low
Prawn, king (jumbo shrimp), plain-cooked	10	1 prawn	2	0	trace	0
Prawn and vegetable stir-fry	250	1 serving	20	30	5	medium
Prawn and avocado sandwiches	454	1 round	11	35	30	medium
Prawn and lettuce sandwiches	347	1 round	10	34	18	medium
Prawn byriani	707	1 serving	11	75	32	medium
Prawn chop suey	225	1 serving	16	34	2	medium
Prawn choux balls	79	1 ball	3	2	8	low
Prawn chow mein	262	1 serving	5	28	1	high

Food	kCalories per portion	Portion size	Protein g	Carbo-hydrate g	Fat g	Fibre
Prawn cocktail	160	1 serving	12	4	9	low
Prawn crackers	44	1 small handful	trace	10	1	low
Prawn curry	220	1 serving	8	36	5	medium
Prawn fajitas	300	2 fajitas	15	34	13	high
Prawn jalfrezi	465	1 serving	26	54	9	high
Prawn mayonnaise sandwiches	513	1 round	10	36	27	medium
Prawn risotto	389	1 serving	47	84	18	low
Prawn rogan josh	562	1 serving	34	17	27	medium
Prawn salad	137	1 serving	26	5	2	high
Prawn salad, dressed	240	1 serving	26	5	13	high
Prawn toast	53	1 toast	2	2	4	low
Prawns (shrimp), canned, drained	80	½ small can	18	0	1	0
Prawns, cooked, peeled	53	2 tablespoons	12	0	1	0
Prawns in garlic butter	284	1 serving	12	trace	24	0
Pretzel flipz	235	1 small bag	4	33	9	low
Pretzels	20	1 small handful	trace	4	trace	low
Prickly pear	42	1 fruit	1	10	trace	high
Processed cheese slice	65	1 slice	4	trace	5	0
Profiteroles with chocolate sauce	373	1 serving	6	33	24	medium
Provolone cheese	99	1 small wedge	7	1	7	0

Food	kCalories per portion	Portion size	Protein g	Carbo- hydrate g	Fat g	Fibre
Prune juice	**136**	1 tumbler	1	36	trace	low
Prunes	**11**	1 prune	trace	3	trace	high
Prunes, canned in natural juice	**79**	3 heaped tablespoons	1	20	trace	high
Prunes, canned in syrup	**90**	3 heaped tablespoons	1	23	trace	high
Ptarmigan, roast	**216**	1 small or ½ large	38	0	8	0
Puffed wheat, dry	**80**	25 g/1 oz/½ cup	4	17	trace	medium
Puffed wheat, with semi-skimmed milk	**185**	5 heaped tablespoons	10	33	2	medium
Puffed wheat, with skimmed milk	**169**	5 heaped tablespoons	10	33	trace	medium
Pumpernickel	**93**	1 slice	3	20	trace	medium
Pumpkin, canned	**34**	3 heaped tablespoons	1	8	trace	medium
Pumpkin, steamed or boiled	**13**	3 heaped tablespoons	1	2	trace	medium
Pumpkin pie	**316**	1 slice	7	41	14	low
Pumpkin seeds	**81**	1 small handful	4	3	7	high
Puri	**328**	1 piece	7	43	25	medium

Prune juice

Puri

Food	kCalories per portion	Portion size	Protein g	Carbo-hydrate g	Fat g	Fibre
Quail, roast	**205**	1 bird	37	0	6	0
Quail's eggs, cooked	**15**	1 egg	1	trace	1	0
Quality street chocolates	**37**	1 sweet (candy)	trace	5	2	0
Quark	**15**	1 tablespoon	2	trace	trace	0
Quarterpounder with cheese	**516**	1 burger in a bun	31	37	27	high
Quavers	**96**	1 small packet	trace	9	6	low
Queen cakes	**245**	1 individual cake	2	26	15	low
Queen of puddings	**341**	1 serving	11	46	13	low
Queen scallops, poached or steamed	**12**	4 scallops	2	0	trace	0
Quenelles, fish	**90**	1 ball/roll	5	3	7	0
Quesadillas	**225**	3 pieces	12	27	9	high
Quiche anglaise	**387**	1 slice	19	17	31	low
Quiche lorraine	**476**	1 slice	23	24	32	low
See also *individual flavours*, e.g. Cheese and onion quiche						
Quince	**17**	1 fruit	trace	4	trace	low
Quince jelly (clear conserve)	**55**	1 tablespoon	trace	13	trace	0
Quinoa	**149**	1 serving	5	28	2	medium
Quinoa porridge, made with semi-skimmed milk	**206**	3 heaped tablespoons	9	34	4	medium
Quinoa porridge, made with skimmed milk	**190**	3 heaped tablespoons	9	34	2	medium

Food	kCalories per portion	Portion size	Protein g	Carbo-hydrate g	Fat g	Fibre
Quinoa porridge, made with water	**149**	3 heaped tablespoons	5	28	2	medium
Quorn, chunks	**74**	1 serving	10	2	3	high
Quorn, fillets	**44**	1 fillet	7	2	1	medium
Quorn, fillets, in breadcrumbs	**185**	1 fillet	10	13	10	high
Quorn, minced (ground)	**79**	1 serving	13	1	3	high
Quorn, sweet and sour	**149**	1 serving	5	29	1	medium
Quorn burger	**117**	1 burger	13	6	5	high
Quorn cottage pie	**212**	1 serving	8	32	6	medium
Quorn fajitas	**303**	2 fajitas	14	45	7	high
Quorn sausages	**115**	1 sausage	13	5	5	high
Quorn southern burgers	**178**	1 burger	11	12	10	high
Quorn spaghetti bolognese	**292**	1 serving	23	38	6	high
Quorn tikka masala, with rice	**540**	1 serving	20	74	21	high

Food	kCalories per portion	Portion size	Protein g	Carbo-hydrate g	Fat g	Fibre
Rabbit and vegetable stew	**404**	1 serving	38	35	3	high
Radicchio	**6**	½ head	trace	1	trace	medium
Radish	**1**	1 radish	trace	trace	trace	low
Radish, winter	**12**	1 radish	1	2	trace	low
Rainbow trout, grilled (broiled)	**240**	1 medium fish	34	0	10	0
Raisin bread	**86**	1 slice	2	15	7	low
Raisin fudge	**87**	1 square	trace	15	2	low
Raisin wheats, dry	**80**	25 g/1 oz/½ cup	2	17	trace	high
Raisin wheats, with semi-skimmed milk	**185**	3 heaped tablespoons	8	34	3	high
Raisin wheats, with skimmed milk	**169**	3 heaped tablespoons	8	34	1	high
Raisins, seedless	**41**	1 small handful	trace	10	trace	high
Raisins, stoned (pitted)	**41**	1 small handful	trace	11	trace	high
Rambutans	**7**	1 fruit	trace	2	trace	low
Rambutans, canned in syrup	**82**	3 heaped tablespoons	1	21	trace	low
Raspberries	**25**	3 heaped tablespoons	1	5	trace	medium
Raspberries, canned in natural juice	**71**	3 heaped tablespoons	1	17	trace	medium
Raspberries, canned in syrup	**88**	3 heaped tablespoons	1	22	trace	medium
Raspberries, stewed	**20**	3 heaped tablespoons	trace	4	trace	medium
Raspberries, stewed with sugar	**48**	3 heaped tablespoons	1	11	trace	medium

Food	kCalories per portion	Portion size	Protein g	Carbo-hydrate g	Fat g	Fibre
Raspberry jam (conserve)	**39**	1 tablespoon	trace	10	0	0
Raspberry milkshake, made with granules See *also* Milkshake	**138**	1 tumbler	6	23	3	low
Raspberry mousse	**137**	1 serving	4	18	6	low
Raspberry pavlova	**320**	1 serving	5	45	14	medium
Raspberry ripple ice cream	**96**	1 scoop	4	12	4	0
Raspberry sauce	**28**	2 tablespoons	trace	7	trace	medium
Raspberry sorbet	**57**	1 scoop	trace	19	trace	low
Raspberry soufflé	**315**	1 serving	6	21	41	0
Raspberry tart	**271**	1 slice	3	24	18	low
Ratafia biscuits (cookies)	**21**	1 biscuit	trace	4	trace	low
Ratatouille	**191**	3 heaped tablespoons	2	11	15	high
Ravioli, dried, boiled	**291**	1 serving	9	45	6	medium
Ravioli, fresh, boiled	**248**	1 serving	12	32	8	medium
Ravioli, in beef and tomato sauce, canned	**154**	½ large can	7	23	5	medium
Ravioli, in tomato sauce, canned	**140**	½ large can	6	20	4	medium
Ray See Skate						
Ready-to-roll icing (frosting)	**96**	25 g/1 oz	0	23	0	0
Ready brek, dry	**89**	25 g/1 oz/½ cup	3	15	2	medium

Food	kCalories per portion	Portion size	Protein g	Carbohydrate g	Fat g	Fibre
Ready brek, with semi-skimmed milk	210	5 heaped tablespoons	9	31	6	high
Ready brek, with skimmed milk	191	5 heaped tablespoons	9	31	3	high
Ready brek, chocolate, dry	90	25 g/1 oz/½ cup	2	16	2	medium
Ready brek, chocolate, with skimmed milk	199	5 heaped tablespoons	9	33	3	high
Ready brek, chocolate, with semi-skimmed milk	215	5 heaped tablespoons	9	33	5	high
Real fruit winders, all flavours	55 (average)	1 roll	trace	11	1	low
Red beet *See Beetroot*						
Red bull	45	1 can	0	11	0	0
Red kidney beans, canned, drained	100	3 heaped tablespoons	7	18	1	high
Red kidney beans, dried, soaked and cooked	103	3 heaped tablespoons	8	17	trace	high
Red leicester cheese	101	1 small wedge	6	trace	8	0
Red salmon *See Salmon*						
Red snapper, baked, stuffed	146	1 medium fish	19	12	2	low
Red snapper, grilled (broiled)	218	1 medium fish	45	0	3	0
Red windsor cheese	100	1 small wedge	6	trace	8	0
Red wine sauce	63	5 tablespoons	1	9	2	0

Food	kCalories per portion	Portion size	Protein g	Carbo-hydrate g	Fat g	Fibre
Redcurrant jelly (clear conserve)	**55**	1 tablespoon	trace	13	trace	0
Redcurrants	**28**	3 heaped tablespoons	1	7	trace	high
Redcurrants, frosted	**27**	1 small bunch	1	7	trace	high
Refried beans	**107**	3 heaped tablespoons	6	15	1	high
Revels	**173**	1 small packet	2	23	6	0
Rhubarb, canned in syrup	**31**	3 heaped tablespoons	trace	8	trace	low
Rhubarb, stewed	**7**	3 heaped tablespoons	1	1	trace	medium
Rhubarb, stewed with sugar	**48**	3 heaped tablespoons	1	11	trace	medium
Rhubarb crumble	**297**	1 serving	3	51	10	medium
Rhubarb fool	**237**	1 serving	5	38	8	medium
Rhubarb pie	**290**	1 slice	3	14	39	medium
Rhubarb sauce	**137**	2 tablespoons	1	34	trace	medium
Ribena, diluted	**103**	1 tumbler	trace	27	0	0
Rice, long-grain, boiled	**248**	1 serving	5	56	2	low
Rice, brown, boiled	**254**	1 serving	5	58	2	medium
Rice, fried (sautéed) See also Egg fried rice and Special fried rice	**236**	1 serving	4	45	6	medium
Rice, savoury	**256**	1 serving	5	47	6	medium
Rice and peas	**247**	1 serving	6	53	3	high
Rice cakes	**35**	1 individual cake	1	7	trace	low
Rice drink	**100**	1 tumbler	trace	20	trace	0

Food	kCalories per portion	Portion size	Protein g	Carbo-hydrate g	Fat g	Fibre
Rice krispies, dry	92	25 g/1 oz/½ cup	1	21	trace	low
Rice krispies, with semi-skimmed milk	205	5 heaped tablespoons	6	40	2	low
Rice krispies, with skimmed milk	189	5 heaped tablespoons	6	40	trace	low
Rice milk	150	300 ml/½ pt/1¼ cups	trace	30	1	0
Rice noodles, boiled	251	1 serving	2	57	trace	low
Rice pudding, canned	323	½ large can	4	43	15	low
Rice pudding, canned, low-fat	136	½ large can	7	23	2	low
Rice pudding, made with semi-skimmed milk	150	1 serving	6	29	2	low
Rice pudding, made with skimmed milk	134	1 serving	6	29	trace	low
Rich tea biscuits (cookies)	39	1 biscuit	1	6	1	low
Ricicles, dry	90	25 g/1 oz/½ cup	1	22.2	0.2	low
Ricicles, with semi-skimmed milk	201	5 heaped tablespoons	4	15	2	low
Ricicles, with skimmed milk	185	5 heaped tablespoons	4	15	trace	low
Ricotta cheese, made with semi-skimmed milk	19	1 tablespoon	1	trace	1	0
Ricotta cheese, whole milk	21	1 tablespoon	1	trace	2	0
Rigatoni (pasta shapes), dried, boiled	198	1 serving	7	42	1	medium
Rigatoni, fresh, boiled	235	1 serving	9	45	2	medium

Food	kCalories per portion	Portion size	Protein g	Carbo-hydrate g	Fat g	Fibre
Ripple chocolate bar	**175**	1 standard bar	3	19	10	0
Risotto See also individual flavours, e.g. Mushroom risotto	**336**	1 serving	4	52	14	low
Risotto, sprinkled with cheese	**449**	1 serving	14	52	22	low
Risotto alla milanese	**403**	1 serving	7	58	18	medium
Rissoles	**134**	1 rissole	5	8	9	low
Ritz original crackers	**17**	1 cracker	trace	1	1	low
Ritz cheese crackers	**17**	1 cracker	trace	1	1	low
Ritz cheese sandwich crackers	**45**	1 sandwich cracker	1	5	2	low
Riva chocolate bar	**136**	1 standard bar	2	14	8	low
Roasted nut cereal bar	**181**	1 bar	3	24	8	medium
Rock cakes	**176**	1 individual cake	3	27	7	low
Rock salmon fried (sautéed), in batter	**580**	1 fillet	30	21	44	low
Rocket	**2**	1 good handful	trace	trace	trace	medium
Rocky chocolate bars, all flavours	**125** (average)	1 standard bar	2	15	7	low
Roes See Cod roes and Herring roes						
Rollmop herring	**180**	1 roll	12	6	12	0
Rolos	**269**	1 tube	2	38	12	0
Romano cheese	**110**	1 small wedge	9	1	8	0

Food	kCalories per portion	Portion size	Protein g	Carbo-hydrate g	Fat g	Fibre
Root beer	135	1 tumbler	0	35	0	0
Roquefort cheese	105	1 small wedge	6	trace	9	0
Rose hip syrup, undiluted	35	1 tablespoon	trace	9	0	0
Roses chocolates	39	1 sweet (candy)	trace	5	2	0
Rosti	156	1 serving	3	25	5	medium
Rotelli (pasta shapes), dried, boiled	198	1 serving	7	42	1	medium
Rotelli, fresh, boiled	235	1 serving	9	45	2	medium
Rouille	151	1 tablespoon	1	2	15	low
Roulade *See individual flavours, e.g.* Chocolate roulade						
Roulé, garlic and herb cheese	77	1 good spoonful	2	1	7	low
Roulé, light	28	1 good spoonful	2	1	2	0
Royal game soup	88	1 serving	5	10	4	low
Royal icing (frosting)	58	1 tablespoon	trace	15	0	0
Rum, dark	55	1 single measure	trace	trace	0	0
Rum, white	55	1 single measure	trace	trace	0	0
Rum and black	123	1 single measure	trace	18	0	0
Rum and coke	94	1 single measure plus 1 mixer	trace	6	0	0
Rum and low-calorie cola	56	1 single measure plus 1 mixer	trace	trace	0	0

Food	kCalories per portion	Portion size	Protein g	Carbo-hydrate g	Fat g	Fibre
Rum and raisin fudge	**87**	1 square	trace	15	2	0
Rum and raisin ice cream	**124**	1 scoop	2	12	4	low
Rum and raisin sauce	**145**	2 tablespoons	1	32	2	low
Rum baba	**326**	1 individual cake	4	47	10	low
Rum butter	**73**	1 tablespoon	trace	8	4	0
Rum punch	**116**	1 wine glass	trace	15	trace	0
Rum sauce, made with semi-skimmed milk	**50**	5 tablespoons	1	5	2	low
Rum sauce, made with skimmed milk	**47**	5 tablespoons	1	5	trace	low
Rump steak See Steak, rump or sirloin						
Runner beans, steamed or boiled	**18**	3 heaped tablespoons	1	2	trace	medium
Ruote (pasta shapes), dried, boiled	**198**	1 serving	7	42	1	medium
Ruote, fresh, boiled	**235**	1 serving	9	45	2	medium
Russian salad	**62**	2 tablespoons	2	5	4	high
Rutabaga See Swede						
Rye bread	**55**	1 medium slice	2	11	trace	medium
Rye bread, light	**35**	1 medium slice	2	12	trace	medium
Ryvita	**27**	1 crispbread	1	5	trace	medium

Food	kCalories per portion	Portion size	Protein g	Carbo-hydrate g	Fat g	Fibre
Sabayon sauce	43	3 heaped tablespoons	1	4	1	0
Sag aloo	163	1 serving	5	21	9	high
Sage derby cheese	101	1 small wedge	6	trace	9	0
Sago pudding, canned	167	½ large can	4	27	7	low
Sago pudding, made with semi-skimmed milk	150	1 serving	6	29	2	low
Sago pudding, made with skimmed milk	134	1 serving	6	29	trace	low
Saint paulin cheese	100	1 small wedge	7	trace	8	0
Saithe See Coley						
Salad cream	52	1 tablespoon	trace	2	5	0
Salad cream, reduced-calorie	29	1 tablespoon	trace	1	2	0
Salade niçoise	308	1 serving	21	34	11	high
Salami, hard-cured	41	1 slice	2	trace	3	0
Salami, moist-cured	57	1 slice	3	trace	5	0
Salmon, baked, stuffed	199	1 steak	26	5	8	low
Salmon, canned, drained	155	½ small can	10	0	4	0
Salmon, grilled (broiled)	367	1 piece of fillet	39	0	25	0
Salmon, in filo pastry (paste)	495	1 portion	42	8	17	low
Salmon, poached or steamed	345	1 piece of fillet	35	0	23	0
Salmon, smoked See also entries for Smoked salmon	119	2 thin slices	21	0	4	0

Food	kCalories per portion	Portion size	Protein g	Carbo-hydrate g	Fat g	Fibre
Salmon, with hollandaise sauce	**559**	1 serving	43	trace	48	0
Salmon and cucumber sandwiches	**378**	1 round	14	35	21	medium
Salmon en croûte	**757**	1 serving	26	46	54	low
Salmon fish cakes, fried (sautéed)	**213**	1 cake	8	15	11	low
Salmon fish cakes, grilled (broiled)	**192**	1 cake	10	17	7	low
Salmon mousse	**205**	1 serving	9	6	6	low
Salmon paste	**33**	1 tablespoon	2	trace	2	0
Salmon pâté	**308**	1 serving	12	0	28	0
Salmon quiche	**363**	1 slice	17	17	25	low
Salmon salad	**376**	1 serving	37	5	24	high
Salmon salad, with mayonnaise	**582**	1 serving	37	5	47	high
Salmon sandwiches	**374**	1 round	14	34	21	medium
Salsa, fresh chilli	**18**	1 tablespoon	trace	4	trace	medium
Salsa, fresh tomato	**14**	1 tablespoon	trace	1	1	medium
Salsify, steamed or boiled	**23**	3 heaped tablespoons	1	9	trace	high
Saltwater crayfish See Dublin bay prawns						
Sambals	**20**	2 tablespoons	1	4	1	medium

Food	kCalories per portion	Portion size	Protein g	Carbo-hydrate g	Fat g	Fibre
Samosa, meat	**300**	1 samosa	2	9	28	low
Samosa, vegetable	236	1 samosa	1	11	21	medium
Sangria	**66**	1 wine glass	trace	4	0	0
Sardine and tomato paste	**23**	1 tablespoon	3	trace	1	0
Sardine pâté	**238**	1 serving	6	0	24	0
Sardines, canned in oil, drained	**108**	½ small can	12	0	7	0
Sardines, canned in tomato sauce	**88**	½ small can	9	trace	6	low
Sardines, canned, on toast	**263**	3 sardines plus 1 slice of toast	15	8	15	low
Sardines, fresh, grilled (broiled)	**67**	1 good-sized fish	7	0	4	0
Satsuma	**23**	1 fruit	trace	5	trace	medium
Sauerkraut, drained	**19**	3 heaped tablespoons	1	4	trace	medium
Sausage and bacon rolls	**105**	1 roll	12	1	24	low
Sausage and egg mcmuffin	**427**	1 portion	23	25	26	medium
Sausage in batter, fried (sautéed)	**235**	1 sausage	7	23	15	low
Sausage mcmuffin	**360**	1 portion	13	26	23	medium
Sausage roll, cocktail	**52**	1 small roll	1	3	1	low
Sausage roll, jumbo	**477**	1 large roll	4	22	24	medium

Food	kCalories per portion	Portion size	Protein g	Carbo-hydrate g	Fat g	Fibre
Sausage roll, puff pastry (paste)	238	1 standard roll	3	16	18	low
Sausage roll, shortcrust pastry (basic pie crust)	229	1 standard roll	4	18	16	low
Sausages See *individual meats, e.g. Pork sausages*						
Savarin	326	1 slice	4	47	10	low
Saveloy	170	1 sausage	6	6	13	low
Savoury rice, cooked	109	1 serving	3	24	0	medium
Scallion *See Spring onion*						
Scallops, fried (sautéed), in breadcrumbs	32	1 scallop	5	1	1	low
Scallops, steamed or poached	12	1 scallop	2	0	trace	0
Scallops mornay	210	1 serving	27	18	3	low
Scaloppine, fried (sautéed), in breadcrumbs	335	1 scallopine	32	20	15	low
Scampi, fried (sautéed), in batter	360	8 pieces	16	24	16	low
Scampi, fried (sautéed), in breadcrumbs	316	8 pieces	12	29	17	low
Scampi provençal	286	1 serving	25	9	10	medium
Schloer	61	1 tumbler	trace	16	0	0
Schnapps	55	1 single measure	trace	trace	0	0

Food	kCalories per portion	Portion size	Protein g	Carbo-hydrate g	Fat g	Fibre
Schnitzel, fried (sautéed), in breadcrumbs	**335**	1 schnitzel	32	20	15	low
Scone (biscuit)	**181**	1 scone	4	27	7	low
Scone, cheese	**175**	1 scone	5	21	9	low
Scone, drop (small pancake)	**44**	1 pancake	1	6	2	low
Scone, fruit	**158**	1 scone	4	26	5	low
Scone, griddle	**44**	1 scone	1	6	2	low
Scone, plain, with butter	**255**	1 scone	4	27	15	low
Scone, plain, with low-fat spread	**220**	1 scone	5	27	11	low
Scone, sweet	**201**	1 scone	4	32	7	low
Scone, sweet, with butter	**275**	1 scone	4	32	15	low
Scone, sweet, with low-fat spread	**240**	1 scone	5	32	11	low
Scone, with clotted cream and jam (conserve)	**308**	1 scone	4	37	16	low
Scotch broth, canned	**88**	2 ladlefuls	4	14	2	medium
Scotch broth, home-made	**156**	2 ladlefuls	12	19	3	high
Scotch egg	**301**	1 egg	14	16	20	low
Scotch pancake	**44**	1 pancake	1	6	2	low
Scotch pie	**225**	1 individual pie	8	24	5	medium
Scotch woodcock	**487**	1 slice	19	18	39	low

Food	kCalories per portion	Portion size	Protein g	Carbo-hydrate g	Fat g	Fibre
Scrambled eggs on toast	**463**	2 eggs plus 1 slice of toast	16	19	37	low
Sea bass, grilled (broiled)	**153**	1 piece of fillet	28	0	4	0
Seafood cocktail	**134**	1 cocktail	6	4	9	low
Seafood enchiladas	**562**	2 enchiladas	32	78	14	medium
Seafood lasagne	**351**	1 serving	22	32	16	high
Seafood pasta	**460**	1 serving	40	62	4	high
Seafood pasta salad	**261**	1 serving	24	29	5	medium
Seafood pizza, thin-crust	**250**	1 slice	12	25	13	medium
Seafood pizza, deep-pan	**315**	1 slice	18	30	15	medium
Seafood salad	**106**	1 serving	17	5	2	high
Seafood salad, with mayonnaise	**312**	1 serving	17	5	24	high
Seafood sticks	**12**	1 stick	2	1	trace	0
Seakale, steamed or boiled	**24**	3 heaped tablespoons	2	1	1	medium
Seaweed	**4**	2 tablespoons	trace	1	trace	low
Seaweed, deep-fried	**131**	3 heaped tablespoons	12	3	12	medium
Seed cake	**423**	1 slice	6	58	20	low
Semolina (cream of wheat), canned	**172**	½ large can	3	27	5	low
Semolina, made with semi-skimmed milk	**150**	1 serving	6	29	2	low

Food	kCalories per portion	Portion size	Protein g	Carbo-hydrate g	Fat g	Fibre
Semolina, made with skimmed milk	134	1 serving	6	29	trace	low
Sesame seeds	90	1 tablespoon	3	trace	9	high
Seven-up	88	1 tumbler	0	22	0	0
Seven-up, diet	3	1 tumbler	0	0	0	0
Seviche	193	1 serving	20	3	18	low
Shandy	48	1 tumbler	trace	13	trace	0
Shark steak, fried (sautéed)	283	1 steak	32	0	13	0
Shark steak, grilled (broiled)	260	1 steak	32	0	8	0
Shark's fin soup	99	2 ladlefuls	7	8	7	0
Sheep's milk	285	300 ml/½ pt/1¼ cups	16	15	18	0
Shepherd's pie	330	1 serving	24	25	19	medium
Sherbert dip	78	1 small packet	0	19	0	0
Sherbert drink	91	1 tumbler	trace	20	1	0
Sherbert fountain	88	1 tube	trace	21	0	0
Sherbert lemons	20	1 sweet (candy)	0	5	0	0
Sherbert oranges	20	1 sweet (candy)	0	5	0	0
Sherbert pips	4	1 pip	0	1	0	0
Sherried chicken	197	¼ small chicken	29	7	4	low
Sherry, dry (fino)	58	1 double measure	trace	1	0	0
Sherry, medium (amontillado)	59	1 double measure	trace	2	0	0
Sherry, sweet (oloroso)	68	1 double measure	trace	3	0	0

Food	kCalories per portion	Portion size	Protein g	Carbo-hydrate g	Fat g	Fibre
Shiitake mushrooms, fresh, fried (sautéed)	**50**	2 tablespoons	1	6	5	low
Shiitake mushrooms, fresh, stewed	**27**	2 tablespoons	1	6	trace	low
Shiitake mushrooms, reconstituted dried, stewed	**35**	1 tablespoon	1	7	trace	low
Shish kebabs	**176**	1 kebab	25	0	8	0
Shortbread fingers	**67**	1 finger	1	8	3	low
Shortcake biscuits (cookies)	**43**	1 biscuit	trace	6	2	low
Shredded wheat, dry	**74**	1 biscuit	2	15	trace	high
Shredded wheat, with semi-skimmed milk	**205**	2 biscuits	9	36	2	high
Shredded wheat, with skimmed milk	**189**	2 biscuits	9	36	1	high
Shredded wheat bitesize, dry	**84**	25 g/1 oz/½ cup	3	17	trace	high
Shredded wheat bitesize, with semi-skimmed milk	**208**	3 heaped tablespoons	9	37	3	high
Shredded wheat bitesize, with skimmed milk	**192**	3 heaped tablespoons	9	37	1	high
Shreddies, dry	**86**	25 g/1 oz/½ cup	2	18	trace	high
Shreddies, with semi-skimmed milk	**213**	5 heaped tablespoons	9	38	3	high
Shreddies, with skimmed milk	**197**	5 heaped tablespoons	9	38	1	high
Shreddies, chocolate, dry	**91**	25 g/1 oz/½ cup	2	20	trace	medium

Food	kCalories per portion	Portion size	Protein g	Carbo- hydrate g	Fat g	Fibre
Shreddies, chocolate, with semi-skimmed milk	224	5 heaped tablespoons	8	42	3	high
Shreddies, chocolate, with skimmed milk	208	5 heaped tablespoons	8	42	1	high
Shreddies, frosted, dry	91	25 g/1 oz/½ cup	2	20	trace	high
Shreddies, frosted, with semi-skimmed milk	224	5 heaped tablespoons	7	43	3	high
Shreddies, frosted, with skimmed milk	208	5 heaped tablespoons	7	43	1	high
Shrimp See Prawns						
Shrimps, canned, drained	80	½ small can	18	0	trace	0
Shrimps, grey or pink, cooked, peeled	15	2 tablespoons	8	0	trace	0
Shrimps, potted	358	1 small pot	16	0	32	0
Shropshire blue cheese	87	1 small wedge	5	trace	7	0
Sieved tomatoes See Passata						
Sild, in oil, drained	108	½ small can	12	0	7	0
Silverskin onions	2	1 onion	trace	trace	trace	low
Simnel cake	298	1 slice	4	49	11	medium
Skate wings, in batter	367	1 wing	33	9	22	low
Skate wings, in black butter	470	1 wing	31	trace	41	0
Skippers, in oil, drained	108	½ small can	12	0	7	0
Skips	87	1 small packet	1	10	5	low

Food	kCalories per portion	Portion size	Protein g	Carbo-hydrate g	Fat g	Fibre
Slivovitz	55	1 single measure	trace	trace	0	0
Sloe gin	35	1 single measure	trace	8	0	0
Smacks, dry	95	25 g/1 oz/½ cup	2	21	trace	low
Smacks, with semi-skimmed milk	209	5 heaped tablespoons	7	40	3	low
Smacks, with skimmed milk	193	5 heaped tablespoons	7	40	1	low
Smarties (M&Ms)	170	1 tube	2	26	9	0
Smelts, fried (sautéed), in seasoned flour	525	5 fish	19	5	47	low
Smoked chicken breast	23	1 slice	2	trace	1	0
Smoked fish *See individual fish, e.g. Salmon, smoked, also Smoked haddock and Smoked salmon*						
Smoked haddock roulade	377	1 serving	30	16	20	low
Smoked pork ring	185	¼ ring	8	1	16	0
Smoked salmon	119	2 thin slices	21	0	4	0
Smoked salmon sandwiches	363	1 round	15	34	19	medium
Smoked salmon and cream cheese bagel	353	1 bagel	17	44	12	medium
Smoked salmon and cream cheese sandwiches	429	1 round	15	34	26	medium
Smoked salmon pâté	273	1 serving	10	0	26	0
Smoked turkey breast	21	1 slice	4	trace	trace	0

Food	kCalories per portion	Portion size	Protein g	Carbo-hydrate g	Fat g	Fibre
Snack shortcake	**40**	1 biscuit (cookie)	trace	5	2	low
Snack wafer bar	**65**	1 finger	trace	7	4	0
Snails, in garlic butter	**311**	6 snails	12	trace	25	low
Snapper, grilled (broiled)	**218**	1 medium fish	45	0	3	0
Snickers chocolate bar	**329**	1 standard bar	6	36	18	low
Snickers ice cream bar	**230**	1 standard bar	4	20	15	low
Snow peas See Mangetout						
Soba noodles, cooked	**228**	1 serving	11	48	trace	high
Soda bread, brown	**80**	1 thick slice	2	15	2	low
Soda bread, white	**82**	1 thick slice	2	12	2	low
Softgrain bread See Bread						
Sole See individual varieties, and cooking methods; e.g. Dover sole, Sole meunière, etc.						
Sole meunière	**376**	1 medium fish	44	trace	22	0
Sole mornay	**243**	1 fillet	47	7	12	low
Sole véronique	**184**	1 fillet	41	11	6	low
Solero ice lolly	**130**	1 lolly	2	20	4	0
Somen noodles, boiled	**230**	1 serving	7	48	trace	medium
Soufflé See individual flavours, e.g. Cheese soufflé						
Soufflé omelette, savoury	**256**	2 eggs	14	trace	22	0

Food	kCalories per portion	Portion size	Protein g	Carbo-hydrate g	Fat g	Fibre
Soufflé omelette, sweet	374	2 eggs	14	10	22	0
Soupe au pistou, canned	60	2 ladlefuls	2	13	1	medium
Soured (dairy sour) cream and chive dressing	38	1 tablespoon	trace	trace	3	low
Soused herring	180	1 roll	12	6	12	0
Soused mackerel	165	1 roll	16	6	9	0
Southern comfort	70	1 single measure	trace	4	0	0
Southern fried chicken	494	2 pieces	36	19	29	low
Soy sauce	10	1 teaspoon	1	1	0	0
Soya beans, canned, drained	140	3 heaped tablespoons	13	5	7	high
Soya beans, dried, soaked and cooked	141	3 heaped tablespoons	14	5	7	high
Soya cheese	106	1 small wedge	6	trace	9	0
Soya cream substitute	28	1 tablespoon	trace	1	3	low
Soya desserts, all flavours	103 (average)	1 individual pot	3	19	2	low
Soya ice desserts, all flavours	44 (average)	1 scoop	trace	5	2	low
Soya milk, sweetened	120	300 ml/½ pt/1¼ cups	9	12	5	low
Soya milk, unsweetened	96	300 ml/½ pt/1¼ cups	9	2	6	low
Soya yoghurt	90	1 individual pot	6	5	5	low
Spaghetti, dried, boiled	239	1 serving	8	51	2	medium

Food	kCalories per portion	Portion size	Protein g	Carbo-hydrate g	Fat g	Fibre
Spaghetti, dried, wholemeal, boiled	**259**	1 serving	31	152	6	high
Spaghetti, fresh, boiled	**301**	1 serving	11	57	2	medium
Spaghetti, with clams	**433**	1 serving	36	52	6	medium
Spaghetti, with meatballs	**718**	1 serving	36	80	31	medium
Spaghetti, with sausages in tomato sauce, canned	**116**	1 small can	8	25	9	medium
Spaghetti, with tomato sauce	**432**	1 serving	12	71	13	high
Spaghetti, with tomato sauce, canned	**128**	1 small can	4	27	1	medium
Spaghetti, with tomato sauce, no-added-sugar, canned-	**101**	1 small can	4	20	1	medium
Spaghetti alfredo	**478**	1 serving	23	67	13	high
Spaghetti bolognese	**456**	1 serving	20	56	19	medium
Spaghetti carbonara	**402**	1 serving	10	56	22	medium
Spaghetti hoops, canned	**122**	1 small can	4	26	1	medium
Spaghetti hoops with hot dogs, canned	**180**	1 small can	6	22	8	low
Spaghetti napoletana	**432**	1 serving	12	71	13	high
Spam	**86**	1 slice	4	trace	8	0
Spanish omelette	**328**	2 eggs	16	17	22	medium
Spanish rice	**228**	1 serving	6	46	2	high
Spare ribs See Pork spare ribs						

Food	kCalories per portion	Portion size	Protein g	Carbo-hydrate g	Fat g	Fibre
Special fried rice	362	1 serving	17	54	9	high
Special K, dry	92	25 g/1 oz/½ cup	4	18	trace	low
Special K, with semi-skimmed milk	205	5 heaped tablespoons	10	36	trace	low
Special K, with skimmed milk	189	5 heaped tablespoons	10	36	trace	low
Special K red berries, dry	92	25 g/1 oz/½ cup	3	18	trace	low
Special K red berries, with semi-skimmed milk	205	5 heaped tablespoons	10	36	2	low
Special K red berries, with skimmed milk	189	5 heaped tablespoons	10	36	trace	low
Spinach	12	1 good handful	1	1	trace	medium
Spinach, cooked	19	3 heaped tablespoons	2	1	1	medium
Spinach, frozen, cooked	21	3 heaped tablespoons	3	trace	1	medium
Spinach and bacon salad	451	1 serving	18	9	44	medium
Spinach roulade	327	1 serving	21	16	20	high
Spinach soup, home-made	132	2 ladlefuls	4	31	trace	medium
Spirali (pasta shapes), dried, boiled	198	1 serving	7	42	1	medium
Spirali, fresh, boiled	235	1 serving	9	45	2	medium
Split pea soup, canned	142	1 serving	8	24	2	high
Split ice lolly, any flavour	83	1 lolly	1	13	3	0
Sponge cake	229	1 slice	3	26	13	low
Sponge cake, fatless	147	1 slice	5	26	3	low

Food	kCalories per portion	Portion size	Protein g	Carbo-hydrate g	Fat g	Fibre
Sponge cake, fatless, filled with cream	343	1 slice	5	36	22	low
Sponge cake, fatless, filled with jam (conserve)	181	1 slice	5	38	3	low
Sponge cake, victoria, filled with cream	490	1 slice	4	52	31	low
Sponge cake, victoria, filled with jam (conserve)	302	1 slice	4	64	5	low
Sponge (lady) fingers	40	1 finger	1	6	1	low
Sporties, dry	89	25 g/1 oz/½ cup	2	19	trace	high
Sporties, with semi-skimmed milk	203	5 heaped tablespoons	8	37	3	high
Sporties, with skimmed milk	187	5 heaped tablespoons	8	37	1	high
Spotted dick	350	1 serving	7	52	16	medium
Sprats, fried (sautéed)	393	5 fish	14	4	35	low
Spring greens (collard greens), steamed or boiled	20	3 heaped tablespoons	2	2	1	medium
Spring onions (scallions)	3	1 onion	trace	trace	trace	low
Spring roll, large	217	1 large roll	7	21	12	low
Spring roll, small	70	1 small roll	3	7	3	low
Spring vegetable soup, canned	62	2 ladlefuls	2	13	trace	medium
Spring vegetable soup, packet	80	2 ladlefuls	2	9	4	low
Sprite	85	1 tumbler	0	22	0	0

Food	kCalories per portion	Portion size	Protein g	Carbo-hydrate g	Fat g	Fibre
Sprite, diet	5	1 tumbler	0	0	0	0
Squab, roast	303	1 bird	37	0	18	0
Squab pie	470	1 serving	40	21	28	medium
Squash *See Marrow*						
Squash, butternut	9	½ medium squash	trace	2	trace	low
Squash, fruit, diluted *See individual flavours, e.g. Orange squash*						
Squid, stewed in olive oil	336	1 serving	13	0	31	0
Squid, stuffed	85	1 squid	6	4	10	low
Squid rings, fried (sautéed), in batter,	235	1 serving	14	19	12	low
Squid risotto	369	1 serving	9	52	15	low
Starfruit	30	1 fruit	trace	7	trace	medium
Starburst sweets (candies)	185	1 tube	trace	38	3	0
Start, dry	90	25 g/1 oz/½ cup	2	20	trace	medium
Start, with semi-skimmed milk	201	5 heaped tablespoons	7	38	3	medium
Start, with skimmed milk	185	5 heaped tablespoons	7	38	1	medium
Steak, fillet, fried (sautéed)	359	1 fillet	48	0	21	0
Steak, fillet, grilled (broiled)	336	1 fillet	48	0	16	0
Steak, rump or sirloin, fried	430	1 steak	50	0	25	0

Food	kCalories per portion	Portion size	Protein g	Carbo-hydrate g	Fat g	Fibre
Steak, rump or sirloin, grilled	381	1 steak	48	0	21	0
Steak and kidney pie	500	1 serving	26	28	32	medium
Steak and kidney pie, individual	484	1 pie	13	38	31	medium
Steak and kidney pudding	431	1 serving	34	24	23	low
Steak and onions	463	1 steak	49	8	27	medium
Steak au poivre	455	1 steak	48	1	29	0
Steak chasseur	417	1 steak	49	7	21	0
Steak diane	488	1 steak	51	3	28	low
Steak sandwiches	685	1 round	53	34	38	low
Steamed sponge pudding	340	1 serving	6	45	16	medium
Steamed suet pudding	221	1 serving	3	34	12	low
Stem lettuce See Chinese leaves						
Sticky toffee pudding	313	1 serving	3	47	12	low
Stifado	565	1 serving	6	45	16	medium
Stilton cheese, blue	103	1 small wedge	6	trace	9	0
Stilton cheese, white	94	1 small wedge	6	trace	8	0
Stock cube, chicken	32	1 cube	1	3	2	0
Stock cube, meat	32	1 cube	1	2	2	0
Stock cube, vegetable	33	1 cube	1	3	2	0
Stollen	177	1 slice	2	26	13	medium

Food	kCalories per portion	Portion size	Protein g	Carbo-hydrate g	Fat g	Fibre
Stout	117	1 small	1	6	trace	0
Straw mushrooms, canned, drained	7	¼ medium can	1	1	trace	0
Strawberries	27	3 heaped tablespoons	1	6	trace	medium
Strawberries, canned in natural juice	48	3 heaped tablespoons	trace	13	trace	medium
Strawberries, canned in syrup	65	3 heaped tablespoons	trace	17	trace	medium
Strawberry cheesecake	296	1 slice	5	32	17	low
Strawberry dessert	101	1 small pot	3	16	3	0
Strawberry ice cream	89	1 scoop	1	12	4	0
Strawberry milkshake, made with granules and semi-skimmed milk	138	1 tumbler	6	23	3	low
Strawberry jam (conserve)	39	1 tablespoon	trace	10	0	0
Strawberry mousse	137	1 serving	4	18	6	low
Strawberry pavlova	320	1 serving	5	45	14	medium
Strawberry shortcake	265	1 serving	5	35	12	low
Strawberry sorbet	57	1 scoop	trace	19	trace	low
Strawberry soufflé	325	1 serving	6	21	41	low
Streusel cake	157	1 slice	3	35	1	low
Striped bass, grilled (broiled)	153	1 piece of fillet	28	0	4	0
Stufato (Italian beef stew)	565	1 serving	6	45	16	medium

Food	kCalories per portion	Portion size	Protein g	Carbo-hydrate g	Fat g	Fibre
Stuffing, made with breadcrumbs and herbs	14	1 tablespoon	trace	3	trace	low
Stuffing, made with rice	31	1 tablespoon	trace	5	1	low
Sugar puffs, dry	97	25 g/1 oz/½ cup	2	22	trace	low
Sugar puffs, with semi-skimmed milk	212	5 heaped tablespoons	7	41	2	low
Sugar puffs, with skimmed milk	196	5 heaped tablespoons	7	41	trace	low
Sugar snap peas	57	10 pods	5	8	1	high
Sugar snap peas, steamed or boiled	52	3 heaped tablespoons	5	7	1	. high
Sugar, all types	20	1 teaspoon	trace	5	trace	0
Sukiyaki	246	1 serving	20	20	9	high
Sultana bran, dry	80	25 g/1 oz/½ cup	2	16	trace	high
Sultana bran, with semi-skimmed milk	185	5 heaped tablespoons	8	33	3	high
Sultana bran, with skimmed milk	169	5 heaped tablespoons	8	33	1	high
Sultana (golden raisin) cake	180	1 slice	2	29	6	medium
Sultanas (golden raisins)	41	1 small handful	trace	10	trace	high
Summer pudding	266	1 serving	7	59	1	high
Sunflower seeds	87	1 tablespoon	4	2	7	high
Supernoodles, all flavours	523 (average)	1 packet	9	67	24	high

Food	kCalories per portion	Portion size	Protein g	Carbo-hydrate g	Fat g	Fibre
Surf 'n' turf	**516**	1 steak plus 2 breaded prawns (shrimp)	51	17	32	low
Sushi	**40**	1 piece	1	8	1	low
Sussex pond pudding	**391**	1 serving	3	50	24	low
Sustain, dry	**90**	25 g/1 oz/½ cup	2	18	1	medium
Sustain, with semi-skimmed milk	**201**	5 heaped tablespoons	8	36	3	medium
Sustain, with skimmed milk	**185**	5 heaped tablespoons	8	36	1	medium
Swede (rutabaga), steamed or boiled	**11**	3 heaped tablespoons	trace	2	trace	low
Sweet and sour chicken	**165**	1 serving	6	32	2	high
Sweet and sour pork	**303**	1 serving	26	31	9	medium
Sweet and sour sauce	**112**	5 tablespoons	trace	16	trace	low
Sweet potatoes, roasted	**190**	4 pieces	2	20	12	medium
Sweet potatoes, steamed or boiled, mashed	**84**	3 heaped tablespoons	1	20	trace	medium
Sweetcorn (corn), kernels, canned	**122**	3 heaped tablespoons	3	27	1	medium
Sweetcorn, on the cob	**99**	1 cob	4	17	2	medium
See *also* Corn cobs *and* Corn on the cob						
Swiss chard, steamed or boiled	**25**	3 heaped tablespoons	2	4	trace	medium

Food	kCalories per portion	Portion size	Protein g	Carbo- hydrate g	Fat g	Fibre
Swiss cheese See also Emmental and Gruyère	107	1 small wedge	8	1	8	0
Swiss cheese fondue	492	1 serving	30	8	29	0
Swiss cheese fondue, with French bread	762	1 serving plus 10 cubes of bread	40	62	31	medium
Swiss (jelly) roll, chocolate	85	1 individual roll	3	14	3	low
Swiss roll, with jam (conserve)	105	1 individual roll	1	24	1	low
Swiss-style muesli See Muesli						
Swordfish steak, fried (sautéed)	294	1 steak	44	0	14	0
Swordfish steak, grilled (broiled)	271	1 steak	44	0	9	0
Syllabub	428	1 serving	1	5	35	0
Syrup, golden (light corn)	45	1 tablespoon	trace	12	0	0
Syrup sauce, for ice cream, bottled, all flavours	92 (average)	2 tablespoons	trace	23	0	0
Syrup sponge pudding	369	1 serving	6	53	16	medium
Syrup tart	368	1 slice	4	60	14	medium

Food	kCalories per portion	Portion size	Protein g	Carbo-hydrate g	Fat g	Fibre
Tabbouleh	**278**	3 heaped tablespoons	7	41	10	high
Taco shell	**57**	1 shell	1	6	3	low
Taco shell, filled with chilli and salad	**170**	1 shell	7	12	10	medium
Tagliarini (pasta strands), dried, boiled	**239**	1 serving	8	51	2	medium
Tagliarini, fresh, boiled	**301**	1 serving	11	57	2	medium
Tagliatelle (pasta ribbons), dried, boiled	**239**	1 serving	8	51	2	medium
Tagliatelle, fresh, boiled	**301**	1 serving	11	57	2	medium
Tahini paste	**91**	1 tablespoon	3	trace	9	medium
Tandoori chicken	**750**	¼ small chicken	95	7	38	low
Tangerine	**44**	1 fruit	1	11	trace	medium
Tangle twister ice lolly	**90**	1 lolly	1	18	2	low
Tango, lemon	**98**	1 tumbler	trace	23	trace	0
See also Apple tango, *etc.*						
Tango, orange	92	1 tumbler	0	25	0	0
Tapioca pudding, canned	**169**	½ large can	3	27	5	low
Tapioca pudding, made with semi-skimmed milk	**150**	1 serving	6	29	2	low
Tapioca pudding, made with skimmed milk	**134**	1 serving	6	29	trace	low
Taramasalata	**223**	2 tablespoons	2	2	23	low

Food	kCalories per portion	Portion size	Protein g	Carbo-hydrate g	Fat g	Fibre
Tartare sauce	43	1 tablespoon	trace	3	3	low
Taxi chocolate bar	134	1 standard bar	1	17	7	low
Tea, black	0	1 cup	trace	trace	trace	0
Tea, with lemon	0	1 cup	trace	trace	trace	0
Tea, with lemon and sugar	20	1 cup plus 1 spoonful of sugar	trace	5	trace	0
Tea, with milk	7	1 cup	trace	trace	1	0
Teacake	180	1 individual teacake	5	32	4	low
Teacake, toasted, with butter	254	1 individual teacake	5	32	12	low
Teacake, toasted, with low-fat spread	219	1 individual teacake	6	32	8	low
Tempura	328	1 serving	23	40	8	low
Tequila	55	1 single measure	trace	trace	0	0
Tequila sunrise	232	1 cocktail	1	24	trace	0
Teriyaki sauce	14	1 tablespoon	trace	3	trace	low
Thai chicken, with noodles	506	1 serving	34	59	15	high
Thai chicken soup	111	2 ladlefuls	3	21	1	low
Thai fragrant rice, steamed or boiled	248	1 serving	5	56	2	low
Thousand island dressing	59	1 tablespoon	trace	2	5	low
Thousand island dressing, low-calorie	12	1 tablespoon	trace	1	1	low
Tia maria	79	1 single measure	trace	6	0	0

Food	kCalories per portion	Portion size	Protein g	Carbo-hydrate g	Fat g	Fibre
Tilsit cheese	**96**	1 small wedge	7	trace	7	0
Time out chocolate bar	**105**	1 finger	1	6	6	low
Tip top topping	**16**	1 tablespoon	1	1	1	low
Tipsy cake	**488**	1 slice	5	41	32	low
Tiramisu	**222**	1 serving	6	24	11	low
Tisanes, all flavours	**0**	1 cup	trace	trace	trace	0
Tizer	**82**	1 tumbler	0	20	trace	low
Tizer, diet	**0**	1 tumbler	0	trace	trace	low
Toad-in-the-hole	**462**	2 thick sausages plus batter	17	33	30	medium
Toast, white, with butter	**155**	1 medium slice	3	18	9	low
Toast, white, with low-fat spread	**120**	1 medium slice	4	18	5	low
Toast, wholemeal, with butter	**153**	1 medium slice	3	15	10	high
Toast, wholemeal, with low-fat spread	**118**	1 medium slice	4	15	6	high
Toasted cheese and ham sandwiches	**438**	1 round	20	36	27	medium
Toffee bon bons	**29**	1 toffee	0	6	1	0
Toffee apple	**251**	1 apple	4	66	trace	high
Toffee crisp chocolate bar	**237**	1 standard bar	2	30	12	low
Toffee fudge ice cream	**90**	1 scoop	1	12	4	0
Toffees, mixed	**20**	1 toffee	trace	1	0	0

Food	kCalories per portion	Portion size	Protein g	Carbo-hydrate g	Fat g	Fibre
Toffos, assorted	**203**	1 tube	1	31	8	0
Tofu, firm	**62**	½ block	8	2	2	low
Tofu, fried (sautéed)	**308**	½ block	20	12	24	medium
Tofu, marinated, baked	**139**	½ block	12	4	10	medium
Tofu, silken	**55**	½ block	5	2	2	low
Tofu, smoked	**148**	½ block	36	1	9	low
Tofu and vegetable stir-fry	**334**	1 serving	17	24	21	high
Tofu burger	**154**	1 burger	10	6	12	medium
Tomato	**13**	1 fruit	1	2	trace	low
Tomato, stuffed, baked	**53**	1 large	3	9	1	medium
Tomato and herb pasta sauce, ready-made	**79**	¼ jar	1	16	trace	low
Tomato and lentil soup, canned	**108**	2 ladlefuls	6	20	trace	medium
Tomato and lentil soup, home-made	**188**	2 ladlefuls	8	26	8	medium
Tomato and lentil soup, instant	**73**	1 mug	3	15	1	low
Tomato and onion salad	**35**	1 serving	2	11	trace	medium
Tomato and onion salad, dressed	**132**	1 serving	2	11	17	medium
Tomato and orange soup, canned	**80**	1 serving	2	17	1	low

Food	kCalories per portion	Portion size	Protein g	Carbo-hydrate g	Fat g	Fibre
Tomato and orange soup, home-made	103	1 serving	2	15	4	medium
Tomato and rice soup, canned	94	1 serving	2	17	2	low
Tomato chutney	24	1 tablespoon	trace	6	trace	low
Tomato juice	28	1 tumbler	2	6	trace	medium
Tomato juice cocktail	36	1 tumbler	2	19	0	low
Tomato ketchup (catsup)	15	1 tablespoon	trace	4	trace	low
Tomato relish	16	1 tablespoon	trace	3	trace	low
Tomato risotto	403	1 serving	7	58	18	medium
Tomato sauce, home-made	67	5 tablespoons	2	6	4	medium
Tomato soup, cream of, canned	110	2 ladlefuls	2	12	7	low
Tomato soup, home-made	86	2 ladlefuls	3	11	4	low
Tomato soup, instant	85	1 mug	1	17	2	medium
Tomato soup, low-fat, canned	50	2 ladlefuls	1	8	1	low
Tomatoes, canned	32	1 small can	2	6	trace	medium
Tomatoes, fried (sautéed)	68	2 halves	trace	4	6	low
Tomatoes, grilled (broiled)	37	2 halves	1	7	1	low
Tomatoes, sieved	29	5 tablespoons	1	6	trace	0
Tomatoes, stewed	25	2 whole	1	4	trace	medium
Tomatoes, sun-dried	5	1 piece	trace	1	trace	low

Food	kCalories per portion	Portion size	Protein g	Carbo-hydrate g	Fat g	Fibre
Tomatoes, sun-dried, in oil, drained	7	1 piece	trace	1	1	low
Tongue, lunch	43	1 slice	1	0	3	0
Tongue, ox, pressed and sliced	73	1 slice	5	0	6	0
Tongue, pork, pressed and sliced	**47**	1 slice	1	0	4	0
Tongues, lambs', canned	213	½ medium can	16	0	16	0
Tonic water	43	1 tumbler	0	10	0	0
Tonic water, low-calorie	4	1 tumbler	trace	0	0	0
Topic chocolate bar	233	1 standard bar	3	27	12	low
Tornado ice cream	**61**	1 ice	0	15	0	0
Tortellini (stuffed pasta), dried, boiled	291	1 serving	9	45	6	medium
Tortellini, fresh, boiled	229	1 serving	9	40	4	medium
Tortilla (spanish omelette)	328	2 eggs	16	17	22	medium
Tortilla chips, all flavours	229	1 small bag	4	30	11	medium
Tortillas, corn	58	1 medium tortilla	1	12	1	medium
Tortillas, flour	159	1 medium tortilla	4	27	3	medium
Tournedos rossini	477	1 fillet steak	52	9	25	low
Tracker bars, all flavours	192 (average)	1 standard bar	3	22	10	medium
Treacle, black (molasses)	38	1 tablespoon	trace	10	0	0
Treacle pudding	369	1 serving	6	53	16	medium

Food	kCalories per portion	Portion size	Protein g	Carbo-hydrate g	Fat g	Fibre
Treacle tart	368	1 slice	4	60	14	medium
Treacle toffee	20	1 piece	trace	1	0	0
Trifle	372	1 serving	10	69	6	high
Trinity cream	453	1 serving	1	15	50	0
Trio chocolate bar	111	1 standard bar	1	12	6	low
Triple chocolate bar	99	1 standard bar	1	12	5	low
Tropical fruit salad	86	3 heaped tablespoons	trace	22	trace	medium
Trout, baked, stuffed	726	1 medium fish	56	41	39	medium
Trout, fried (sautéed)	232	1 medium fish	33	0	13	0
Trout, grilled (broiled)	209	1 medium fish	33	0	8	0
Trout, poached or steamed	200	1 medium fish	35	0	7	0
Trout, smoked	136	1 fillet	23	0	5	0
Trout, smoked, pâté	269	1 serving	11	0	24	0
Trout meunière	388	1 medium fish	46	trace	29	0
Trout with almonds	464	1 medium fish	48	1	36	medium
Truffles	50	1 truffle	1	6	2	low
Truite au bleu	200	1 medium fish	35	0	7	0
Tuc crackers	25	1 cracker	trace	3	1	low
Tuc savoury sandwiches	76	1 sandwich	1	7	5	low
Tuna, canned in brine, drained	107	½ standard can	23	0	trace	0
Tuna, canned in oil, drained	182	½ standard can	27	0	7	0

Food	kCalories per portion	Portion size	Protein g	Carbo-hydrate g	Fat g	Fibre
Tuna and cucumber sandwiches	**352**	1 round	15	35	18	medium
Tuna and pasta casserole	**285**	1 serving	22	30	9	medium
Tuna and sweetcorn pasta	**451**	1 serving	37	50	11	medium
Tuna mornay	**241**	1 serving	29	7	10	low
Tuna mousse	**185**	1 serving	11	6	10	low
Tuna salad	**138**	1 serving	25	5	1	high
Tuna salad, with mayonnaise	**344**	1 serving	25	11	23	high
Tuna steak, fried (sautéed)	**345**	1 steak	52	0	15	0
Tuna steak, grilled (broiled)	**322**	1 steak	52	0	10	0
Tunes sweets (candies)	**145**	1 tube	0	36	0	0
Turbot, grilled (broiled)	**194**	1 piece of fillet	33	0	6	0
Turbot, steamed or poached	**159**	1 piece of fillet	36	0	1	0
Turkey, breast, smoked	**21**	1 slice	4	trace	trace	0
Turkey, fillets, fried (sautéed)	**248**	1 medium fillet	40	3	9	0
Turkey fillets, grilled (broiled)	**225**	1 medium fillet	40	3	4	0
Turkey fillets, fried, in breadcrumbs	**326**	1 medium fillet	43	13	9	low
Turkey, minced (ground), stewed	**197**	1 serving	31	0	5	0
Turkey, roast, with skin	**171**	2 medium slices	28	0	6	0
Turkey, roast, without skin	**140**	2 medium slices	29	0	3	0

Food	kCalories per portion	Portion size	Protein g	Carbo-hydrate g	Fat g	Fibre
Turkey, roast, with stuffing and sausagemeat	229	1 serving	33	12	5	medium
Turkey and vegetable casserole	298	1 serving	23	32	8	medium
Turkey and vegetable soup, home-made	134	2 ladlefuls	10	14	4	medium
Turkey and vegetable stir-fry	259	1 serving	29	31	3	high
Turkey bacon, grilled (broiled)	34	1 slice	2	trace	3	0
Turkey burger in a bun, with relish, home-made	357	1 burger in a bun	38	32	9	low
Turkey fingers, fried (sautéed), in batter or breadcrumbs	178	1 finger	9	11	11	low
Turkey ham	36	1 slice	5	trace	1	0
Turkey pot pie	485	1 slice	17	28	39	low
Turkey roll	41	1 slice	5	trace	2	0
Turkey sandwiches	345	1 round	10	34	19	medium
Turkey soup, home-made	111	2 ladlefuls	13	7	2	0
Turkey stew	430	1 serving	34	65	3	medium
Turkish delight, chocolate covered-	185	1 standard bar	1	37	4	0
Turkish delight, in icing (confectioners') sugar	29	1 cube	trace	8	0	0

Food	kCalories per portion	Portion size	Protein g	Carbo-hydrate g	Fat g	Fibre
Turnips, glazed	**55**	3 heaped tablespoons	1	15	trace	medium
Turnips, steamed or boiled	**12**	3 heaped tablespoons	1	2	trace	medium
Tuscan bean salad	**120**	3 heaped tablespoons	4	12	5	high
Tutti frutti ice cream	**75**	1 scoop	1	5	7	low
Twiglets	**136**	1 small bag	4	16	3	medium
Twirl chocolate bar	**115**	1 finger	2	12	7	0
Twistetti (pasta shapes), dried, boiled	**198**	1 serving	7	42	1	medium
Twistetti, fresh, boiled	**235**	1 serving	9	45	2	medium
Twix chocolate bar	**143**	1 finger	2	18	7	low
Twix ice cream	**228**	1 standard bar	3	23	14	low
Tzatziki	**20**	2 tablespoons	1	1	1	low

Food	kCalories per portion	Portion size	Protein g	Carbo-hydrate g	Fat g	Fibre
Vacherin, with cream and fruit	**320**	1 slice	5	45	14	medium
Vanilla fudge	**77**	1 square	trace	14	2	0
Vanilla cheesecake	**490**	1 slice	4	30	27	low
Vanilla ice cream, dairy	**97**	1 scoop	2	12	5	0
Vanilla ice cream, non-dairy	**89**	1 scoop	2	11	4	0
Vanilla soufflé	**236**	1 serving	7	26	1	low
Veal, cutlet, fried (sautéed), in breadcrumbs	**376**	1 cutlet	55	8	14	low
Veal, cutlet, grilled (broiled)	**300**	1 cutlet	52	0	9	0
Veal, escalope, fried, in breadcrumbs	**335**	1 escalope	32	20	15	low
Veal, roast	**230**	2 thick slices	32	0	11	0
Veal birds	**450**	2 rolls	52	12	20	low
Veal fricassée	**339**	1 serving	27	34	9	low
Vegemite	**8**	1 teaspoon	1	trace	0	0
Vegetable bake	**360**	1 serving	12	33	10	high
Vegetable casserole	**228**	1 serving	12	33	6	high
Vegetable cottage pie	**350**	1 serving	15	48	12	high
Vegetable curry	**183**	1 serving	5	34	4	high
Vegetable deluxe burger	**423**	1 burger in a bun	10	54	18	high
Vegetable goulash	**338**	1 serving	12	142	15	high
Vegetable juice	**41**	1 tumbler	trace	9	trace	0

Food	kCalories per portion	Portion size	Protein g	Carbo-hydrate g	Fat g	Fibre
Vegetable lasagne	424	1 serving	15	50	10	high
Vegetable pâté	138	1 serving	10	1	10	low
Vegetable pie	425	1 individual pie	6	52	23	medium
Vegetable risotto	372	1 serving	6	58	15	low
Vegetable samosa	236	1 samosa	1	11	21	medium
Vegetable soup, canned	74	2 ladlefuls	3	13	1	high
Vegetable soup, home-made	93	2 ladlefuls	3	4	trace	high
Vegetable soup, packet	46	2 ladlefuls	2	8	1	low
Vegetable stew	186	1 serving	7	31	4	high
Vegetable stir-fry	169	1 serving	7	15	6	high
Vegetable terrine	155	1 thick slice	8	17	7	high
Vegetables, mixed, canned, drained	38	3 heaped tablespoons	2	6	1	medium
Vegetables, mixed, frozen, cooked	42	3 heaped tablespoons	3	7	trace	high
Veggie burger	85	1 burger	7	5	4	medium
Veggie sausage	75	1 sausage	3	6	4	medium
Velouté sauce	99	5 tablespoons	1	4	9	low
Venison, roast	198	2 thick slices	35	0	6	0
Venison, stewed	225	1 serving	25	8	7	low
Vermicelli (pasta strands), dried, boiled	239	1 serving	8	51	2	medium
Vermicelli, fresh, boiled	301	1 serving	11	57	2	medium

Food	kCalories per portion	Portion size	Protein g	Carbo-hydrate g	Fat g	Fibre
Vermouth, bianco	67	1 double measure	trace	8	0	0
Vermouth, extra dry	59	1 double measure	trace	3	0	0
Vermouth, red	75	1 double measure	trace	8	0	0
Vermouth, rosso	85	1 double measure	trace	8	0	0
Vichyssoise, canned	108	2 ladlefuls	2	12	6	low
Vichyssoise, home-made	117	2 ladlefuls	2	8	6	low
Victoria sandwich, filled with jam (conserve)	302	1 slice	4	64	5	low
Viennetta, all flavours	227 (average)	1 slice	3	23	14	0
Vienna bread	109	1 thick slice	3	15	1	low
Viennese finger, filled	81	1 biscuit (cookie)	1	9	5	low
Vimto	52	1 tumbler	trace	20	trace	0
Vinaigrette dressing	101	1 tablespoon	trace	trace	11	0
Vinaigrette dressing, low-calorie	5	1 tablespoon	trace	1	trace	0
Vine leaves, stuffed	221	2 rolls	18	19	9	high
Vinegar, all types	1	1 tablespoon	trace	trace	0	0
Vitbe bread	82	1 medium slice	3	16	1	medium
Vitello tonnato	594	1 escalope	44	20	37	low
Vodka	55	1 single measure	trace	trace	0	0
Vodka and orange	108	1 single measure	trace	7	0	0

Food	kCalories per portion	Portion size	Protein g	Carbo-hydrate g	Fat g	Fibre
Vodka and tonic	76	1 single measure plus 1 mixer	trace	5	0	0
Vodka and tonic, low-calorie	58	1 single measure plus 1 mixer	trace	trace	trace	0
Vodka martini	114	1 cocktail	trace	3	trace	0
Vol-au-vents, all flavours	286 (average)	1 medium	11	20	18	low
Vol-au-vents, cocktail, all flavours	143 (average)	1 small	5	10	9	low

Food	kCalories per portion	Portion size	Protein g	Carbo-hydrate g	Fat g	Fibre
Wafer biscuits (cookies), chocolate-covered	115	1 biscuit	1	13	6	low
Wafer biscuits, filled	39	1 biscuit	1	7	2	low
Wafers, for ice cream	17	1 wafer	2	4	trace	low
Waffle, potato, fried (sautéed) or baked	84	1 waffle	1	13	3	low
Waffle, sweet	240	1 waffle	8	30	8	low
Waffles, sweet, with maple syrup	533	2 waffles	16	75	16	medium
Waffles, with bacon and maple syrup	799	2 waffles plus 2 rashers (slices) of bacon	36	75	48	medium
Walnut cake	344	1 slice	7	34	19	medium
Walnut whip	165	1 whip	7	20	8	low
Walnut whirl, chocolate	20	1 chocolate	trace	2	1	low
Walnuts, shelled	172	25 g/1 oz/¼ cup	4	1	17	high
Water biscuits (crackers)	33	1 biscuit	1	6	1	low
Water chestnuts, canned, drained	14	4 pieces	trace	3	trace	low
Watercress	3	1 good handful	trace	trace	trace	medium
Watercress soup	99	2 ladlefuls	1	14	2	low
Watermelon	66	1 large wedge	1	14	1	low
Weetabix, dry	64	1 biscuit	2	13	trace	high

Food	kCalories per portion	Portion size	Protein g	Carbo- hydrate g	Fat g	Fibre
Weetabix, with semi-skimmed milk	169	2 biscuits	8	32	trace	high
Weetabix, with skimmed milk	185	2 biscuits	8	32	2	high
Weetaflakes, dry	90	25 g/1 oz/½ cup	2	20	1	high
Weetaflakes, with semi skimmed milk-	201	5 heaped tablespoons	8	38	3	high
Weetaflakes, with skimmed milk	185	5 heaped tablespoons	8	38	1	high
Weetos, dry	96	25 g/1 oz/½ cup	1	20	1	medium
Weetos, with semi-skimmed milk	172	5 heaped tablespoons	6	30	4	medium
Weetos, with skimmed milk	154	5 heaped tablespoons	6	30	2	medium
Welsh rarebit	242	1 slice	10	21	13	low
Wensleydale cheese	94	1 small wedge	6	trace	8	0
Westphalian ham	29	1 slice	4	trace	2	0
Wheat bran	31	1 tablespoon	2	4	1	high
Wheat crunchies, all flavours	180 (average)	1 small packet	4	20	9	low
Whelks, boiled	14	1 serving	3	trace	trace	0
Whippy ice cream	85	1 cornet	2	12	3	low
Whisky	55	1 single measure	trace	trace	0	0

Food	kCalories per portion	Portion size	Protein g	Carbo-hydrate g	Fat g	Fibre
Whisky and coke	99	1 single measure plus 1 mixer	trace	6	0	0
Whisky and coke, low-calorie	56	1 single measure plus 1 mixer	trace	trace	trace	0
Whisky and ginger ale	75	1 single measure plus 1 mixer	trace	5	0	0
Whisky and ginger ale, low-calorie	55	1 single measure plus 1 tumbler	trace	trace	0	0
Whisky mac	255	1 single measure plus 1 double measure	trace	trace	0	0
Whisky sour	157	1 cocktail	0	14	0	0
White pudding, fried (sautéed) or baked	450	2 thick slices	7	36	32	low
White sauce, savoury, made with semi-skimmed milk	96	5 tablespoons	3	8	6	low
White sauce, savoury, made with skimmed milk	86	5 tablespoons	3	8	5	low
White sauce, sweet, made with semi-skimmed milk	112	5 tablespoons	3	14	5	low
White sauce, sweet, made with skimmed milk	92	5 tablespoons	3	14	4	low
White stilton cheese	94	1 small wedge	6	trace	8	0
White wine sauce	75	1 serving	2	6	2	low
Whitebait, fried (sautéed)	525	1 serving	19	5	47	low

Food	kCalories per portion	Portion size	Protein g	Carbo-hydrate g	Fat g	Fibre
Whiting, fried (sautéed), in breadcrumbs	334	1 fillet	31	12	17	low
Whiting, poached or steamed	110	1 fillet	24	0	1	0
Whiting, smoked, poached	166	1 fillet	25	1	1	0
Wholegrain mustard	7	1 teaspoon	2	1	trace	low
Wholenut chocolate bar	270	1 standard bar	5	24	17	medium
Whopper	660	1 burger	29	47	40	high
Whopper, with cheese	760	1 burger	35	47	48	high
Whopper, double	920	2 burgers	49	47	21	high
Whopper, double, with cheese	1010	2 burgers	55	47	67	high
Wiener schnitzel	335	1 schnitzel	32	20	15	low
Wild rice, cooked	182	1 serving	7	6	trace	0
Wild rice mix, cooked	177	1 serving	6	31	1	low
Winders, real fruit	55	1 roll	trace	11	1	low
Wine gums	119	1 tube	3	27	trace	0
Wine, dry white, sparkling	95	1 wine glass	trace	2	0	0
Wine, dry white	82	1 wine glass	trace	1	0	0
Wine, low-alcohol, red	70	1 wine glass	trace	2	0	0
Wine, low-alcohol, rosé	70	1 wine glass	trace	2	0	0
Wine, low-alcohol, white	70	1 wine glass	trace	2	0	0
Wine, medium white	94	1 wine glass	trace	4	0	0
Wine, mulled	105	1 wine glass	trace	5	0	0

Food	kCalories per portion	Portion size	Protein g	Carbo-hydrate g	Fat g	Fibre
Wine, red	85	1 wine glass	trace	0	trace	0
Wine, rosé	89	1 wine glass	trace	1	0	0
Wine, sweet	117	1 wine glass	trace	7	0	0
Winkles	14	1 serving	3	trace	trace	0
Winter radish	12	1 radish	1	2	trace	low
Wispa chocolate bar	210	1 standard bar	3	21	13	0
Wispa, gold	265	1 standard bar	3	29	15	0
Wispa, mint	275	1 standard bar	3	27	17	0
Witch, fried (sautéed), in breadcrumbs	342	1 medium fish	25	15	21	low
Witch, grilled (broiled)	158	1 medium fish	25	0	4	0
Witch, poached or steamed	112	1 medium fish	25	0	1	0
Woodcock, roast	303	1 bird	37	0	18	0
Worcestershire sauce	17	1 tablespoon	trace	4	0	0
Wotsits, all flavours	115 (average)	1 small packet	2	12	7	low

Food	kCalories per portion	Portion size	Protein g	Carbo-hydrate g	Fat g	Fibre
Yam, roast	**156**	4 pieces	2	33	5	medium
Yam, steamed or boiled, mashed	**133**	3 heaped tablespoons	2	33	trace	medium
Yeast extract	**9**	1 teaspoon	2	trace	trace	0
Yellow bean sauce	**19**	1 tablespoon	trace	4	trace	low
Yellow beans, fresh, steamed or boiled	**25**	3 heaped tablespoons	2	5	trace	high
Yellow melon	**63**	1 large wedge	1	15	trace	medium
Yoghurt (plain)	**99**	1 individual pot	7	10	4	0
Yoghurt, all flavours	**131** (average)	1 individual pot	6	20	4	0
Yoghurt, bio	**56**	1 small pot	5	7	1	0
Yoghurt, custard-style	**161**	1 small pot	8	3	13	0
Yoghurt, drinking	**124**	1 tumbler	6	26	trace	0
Yoghurt, fruit corner	**219**	1 individual carton	6	26	7	low
Yoghurt, greek-style, cows'	**161**	1 individual pot	8	3	13	0
Yoghurt, greek-style, sheep's	**149**	1 individual pot	6	8	10	0
Yoghurt, low-calorie, plain	**51**	1 individual pot	5	7	trace	0
Yoghurt, low-fat, plain	**70**	1 individual pot	6	9	1	0
Yoghurt, low-fat, all flavours	**112** (average)	1 individual pot	5	22	1	0
Yoghurt, soya	**90**	1 individual pot	6	5	5	0

Food	kCalories per portion	Portion size	Protein g	Carbo-hydrate g	Fat g	Fibre
Yoghurt ice-cream, all flavours	**53** (average)	1 scoop	3	8	1	low
Yoghurt jelly (jello), made with plain, low-fat yoghurt	**60**	1 serving	5	12	1	0
Yorkie bar, milk	**317**	1 standard bar	4	35	18	0
Yorkie bar, nut	**312**	1 standard bar	6	26	10	low
Yorkie bar, raisin and biscuit (cookie)	**265**	1 standard bar	3	32	13	low
Yorkshire parkin	**185**	1 piece	2	29	7	low
Yorkshire pudding	**62**	1 small pudding	2	7	3	low

Food	kCalories per portion	Portion size	Protein g	Carbo-hydrate g	Fat g	Fibre
Zabaglione	**87**	1 serving	3	8	3	0
Zite (pasta shapes), dried, boiled	**198**	1 serving	7	42	1	medium
Zite, fresh, boiled	**235**	1 serving	9	45	2	medium
Zoom ice lolly	**46**	1 lolly	trace	10	trace	0
Zucchini See Courgettes						